Hildegard of Bingen's
MEDICINE

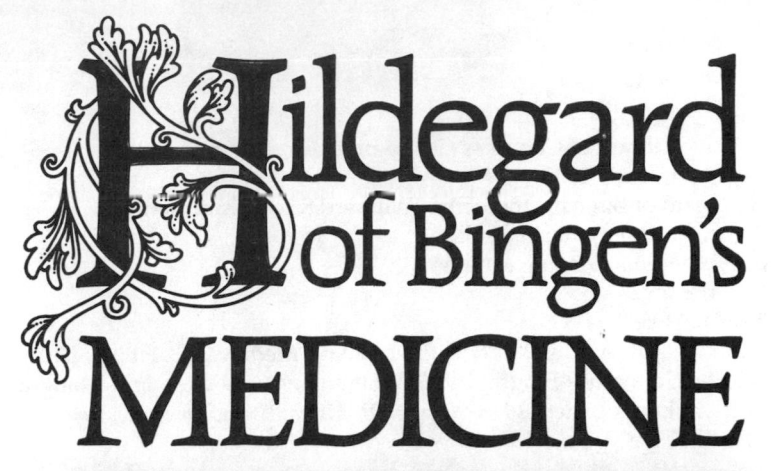

MEDICINE

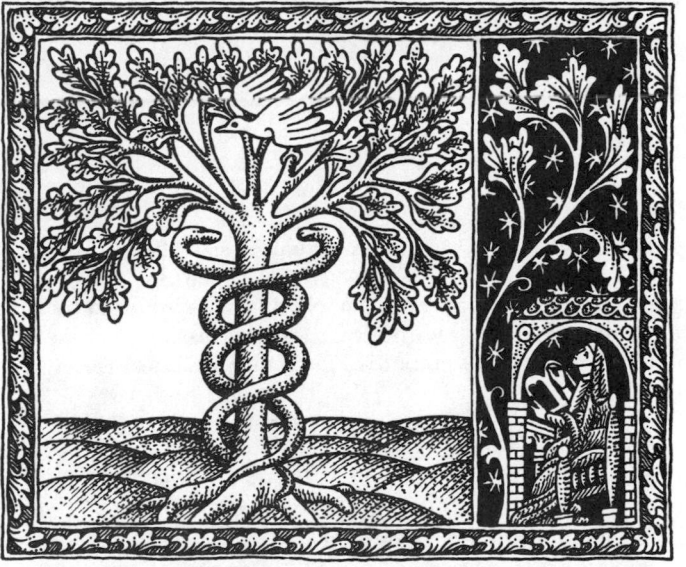

Dr. Wighard Strehlow & Gottfried Hertzka, M.D.

translated from the German by
Karin Anderson Strehlow

BEAR & COMPANY
SANTA FE, NEW MEXICO

Library of Congress Cataloging-in-Publication Data
Strehlow, Wighard, 1937-
Hildegard of Bingen's medicine/Wighard Srtehlow & Gottfried
Hertka; translated by Karin Strehlow.
p.   cm.-(Folk wisdom series)
Includes index.
ISBN 0-939680-44-0
1. Hildegard, Saint. 1098-1179. 2. Medicine, Medieval. 3. Homeopathy.
4. Healers—Germany—Biography. 5. Women mystics—Germany—Biogra-
phy. I. Hertzka, Gottfried. 1913-   II. Title. III. Series.
R144.H54S77 1987
615.8'82—dc19   87-27306
                                                                 CIP

Bear & Company, Inc.
Santa Fe, NM 87504-2860

Editor: Gail Vivino
Cover Illustration: Copyright © 1988 Angela C. Werneke
Design: Angela C. Werneke

Hildegard illuminations in text are from *Hildegard of Bingen's Scivias* and *Hildegard of
Bingen's Book of Divine Works*, illustrated by Angela C. Werneke and published by Bear
& Company. Ornamental initials and vignettes, with minor modification, are from
Historic Alphabets and Initials, edited by Carol Belanger Grafton and published by
Dover Publications, Inc. Cover illustration by Angela C. Werneke.

Printed in the United States of America by BookCrafters, Inc.

9 8 7 6

This book is dedicated to Punkie
who translated Hildegard's poetic language
into English.

EDITOR'S NOTE

Many translated excerpts from Hildegard of Bingen's original writings will be found throughout this book. To set them apart from the remaining majority of the text by Drs. Hertzka and Strehlow, these excerpts from Hildegard have all been set in italic type. It should be noted that occasionally, within these excerpts, there is a notation or comment contained in brackets. This bracketed material is not original Hildegard text, but is experienced opinion or commentary inserted by Drs. Hertzka and Strehlow.

Note also that Bear & Company, the publisher of this book, does not support the use of products which in any way threaten the survival of endangered or precious species on this planet. The use of substances such as whale meat, ivory powder, or vulture beak powder, as mentioned in this book, is solely up to the discretion of the reader.

Readers wishing to study this book in the German from which this English edition was translated will find it under the title, *Handbuch der Hildegard-Medizin*, published in 1987 by Berlag Hermann Bauer, Freiburg im Breisgau, Germany.

G.V.

CONTENTS

SPECIAL NOTICE TO
THE READER

This book is a reference work and as such is intended solely for use as a source of general information and not for application to any individual case. It is based on the divinely inspired writings of the twelfth-century mystic, Hildegard of Bingen, and on the interpretations, opinions, and experiences with these writings of the physicians who are the authors of this book. The authors and publisher have made every effort to correctly interpret and translate the original intentions of this material, which was first written in twelfth-century Middle Latin language, later translated into German, and then translated into twentieth-century English. It should be noted, however, that the opinions expressed herein are not necessarily those of, nor endorsed by, the publisher; nor can the publisher certify that use of the procedures, recommendations, or substances contained herein is safe or will produce the results described in each individual case.

The information contained in the following pages is in no way to be considered as a substitute for consultation, diagnosis, and/or treatment by a duly licensed physician or other health-care professional. Such professionals are in a position to evaluate an individual case and suggest appropriate measures dependent on the circumstances.

FOREWORD

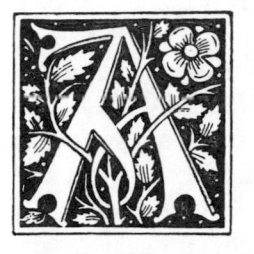s a practitioner of herbal medicine for over fifteen years, I have studied in depth the energetic systems of Oriental medicine, including both the Chinese and the Ayurvedic of India. While I have studied Western herbalism as well, I found the lack of such an energetic system with its more organic differentiation of herbs and diseases to greatly limit its effectiveness. It thereby became my concern to bring back such a system into Western herbalism. Systems which organize medicines and diseases according to prime elements, energies, and biological humors reflect the language of nature and are more effective in transmitting nature's healing power. Such systems did exist in ancient and medieval Western medicine. Fragments of them endured into the early part of this century. Though once common, their traces have largely been eradicated and discredited by allopathic medicine. Now that the limitations of allopathy are clear to many of us, the validity of these traditional systems is again becoming apparent.

Reliable and practical knowledge of these older Western systems is hard to find. Saint Hildegard of Bingen, a German mystic of the twelfth century, gives us in her work such precious knowledge, much of which is as applicable today as it was in her lifetime centuries ago. Hildegard uses the four-element system and the four-humor system, which date back at least to the time of the ancient Greeks. This model had a strong effect on middle-eastern or Islamic medicine and has much in common with the humoral and elemental system of Ayurveda, the traditional medicine of India. By bringing us back to this organic model, her knowledge can help Western herbal medicine return itself to an equal level of sophistication with the Eastern systems that are becoming popular today. Hildegard's medicine, therefore, has a special import today for this regeneration of our own older natural-healing tradition.

In addition, Hildegard integrates natural medicine with spiritual knowledge. Hildegard was primarily a mystic concerned with our relationship with the Divine. She produced many religious, philosophical, and devotional works. Her medical knowledge was a facet of her greater spiritual work. She reveals an understanding of the complete nature of the human being and sets forth a comprehensive system of healing for body, mind, and spirit. As such, her medicine is part of a total healing system. It is this integration of physical healing with psychological and spiritual healing that alone is truly holistic and which many of us today are seeking in terms of holistic health. Hildegard's wisdom will be helpful towards this aim as well. Her language may be easier to understand for those of a Western or Christian background who find the holistic systems of the East interesting but difficult to fit into. Even those of us who do not share her Christian language or that of the authors of this book will find in her medicine much knowledge of natural healing that is universally applicable, which we will be able to extract and use in our own way.

She not only tells us much about herbs and foods but also much about the disharmony of elements responsible for disease and the underlying disharmony of the soul. She indicates the conditions of body and mind that reflect the imbalance of natural humors. For example, she ascribes many diseases to the accumulation of black bile, which is very similar to suppressed emotions. What she offers, therefore, is not just remedies but a system of diagnosis and an understanding of the disease process, which itself indicates the appropriate means of restoring balance. Her diagnosis through examination of the eyes, which starts out the book, is particularly informative. The eyes as the mirror of the soul reflect the true essence of both our spirit and our vitality.

Hildegard produced all of her works, as she has said, through her heavenly or spiritual vision. She did not rely on medical experience or upon traditional learning; nevertheless her healing system is practical and valid. In this regard, she teaches us that we have an inner wisdom that is more sophisticated than profound outer study and experience. If we relied more on that today, we would undoubtedly have better healers. As it is, we sharpen our surgical tools, refine our drugs, and do massive testing, but are we really any closer to the heart of creation and the real power of life? We gain more information and accumulate more licenses and titles for ourselves and are still confused as to what real health is or as to the real purpose of human life, which has to be something more than the accumulation of mere things. Hildegard shows us the direction to which we need to return. True healing cannot be arrived at by outer action alone; it requires contacting that inner consciousness and organic intelligence which is the real healing power. This, as her writings indicate, is an act of faith; it cannot be done mechanically or merely intellectually. It requires opening up to the spiritual force in us and in the world around us. In that alone is the real root of medicine, not in hospitals or medical colleges.

Many of Hildegard's remedies reflect a knowledge that is found in other herbal systems. It is not only consistent with most of later Western herbalism, it is also often similar to that of such Eastern systems as Ayurveda or traditional Chinese medicine. She uses psyllium for constipation, just as later Western herbalists do; aloe for jaundice; and horehound for cough. Many other such examples could be cited. She employs herbs from the East as well as the West. Some of her favorite remedies are spices from the Orient. One such herb she uses frequently is galangal (*Alpinia galanga*), a ginger relative. To this herb, long used for the treatment of indigestion, stomach pain, and arthritic pain, she attributes the power to stop heart pain and revive the heart, similar to the effects of nitroglycerine. As the authors state, "If there would be a drug to wake up the dead, then galangal would be the first choice." Hildegard also has some special or uncommonly used remedies like geranium for colds and columbine for scrofula, giving us new knowledge on these herbs.

Many of her remedies are common herbs, like fennel, parsley, and nettles, which can be found almost everywhere. She often gives simple home or kitchen remedies, like parsley wine. As such, her prescriptions can be used for many general conditions as part of self-healing and family care without the need for more sophisticated diagnoses. Most of Hildegard's remedies are easy to prepare and consist of few ingredients. They consist of many different preparations including herbal teas, wines, syrups, oils, salves, powders, and smoking mixtures. In addition, she prepares herbs with foods like herbal eggs or herbal cookies.

Like the medieval alchemists with whom she has much in common, Hildegard integrates the use of gems and minerals into her usage of herbs. She recommends such remedies as gold for arthritis, emerald for heart pain, jasper for hay fever or for cardiac arrhythmia, gold topaz for loss of vision, and blue sapphire for eye inflammation. She uses gem wines, similar to the gem tinctures now being used more widely today. The qualities she ascribes to gems are very similar to those given to them in Ayurvedic medicine. She also uses some animal parts. In all of this, is not medieval superstition but an understanding of healing substances which extends to the whole of nature and can be verified by the experience in traditional healing systems throughout the world? It is interesting to see such a profound healing system using such a wide variety of substances, some from distant lands, in what were supposed to be the dark ages. Many of us today are just beginning to integrate such different healing substances, like herbs and gems, and Hildegard provides a helpful foundation to work with in this regard.

Diet is also essential to her healing system and she sets forth sound principles for a balanced diet. She speaks of the danger of too much cold or raw food, which can weaken the digestive fire, just as she does of the danger of too much meat or fat. Hildegard's dietary approach exposes both the excesses of the heavy meat-eating of most Westerners, and also shows those that can occur by some of the extreme natural-food proponents. Her diet, which includes some meat and much seafood, along with vegetables and grains (spelt, a kind of wheat, is her favorite) is one that is not too difficult to follow. She prescribes beer and wine under certain conditions as well. She has many interesting and provocative observations about different foods and their qualities, which any nutritionist should examine. In this regard, she explains the chestnut as the ideal food for the brain and nerves.

Hildegard employs other healing methods, including fasting, bloodletting, cupping, and saunas. Bloodletting, more accurately styled therapeutic release of toxic blood, is an effective cleansing method that deserves wider examination. Her exposition of these methods adds new insight into their application.

The German authors of this book have extracted from Hildegard's works her medical knowledge and have organized it in a cogent manner. They examine many modern illnesses in light of Hildegard's medicine and add their own voice and knowledge to show its continued relevance. They regard Hildegard with much enthusiasm as a source of divine wisdom, and it is the extensive quotes from her writings that are the highlight of this book. Dr. Gottfried Hertzka is a medical doctor and Dr. Wighard Strehlow was a research chemist in the pharmaceutical industry in West Germany until he became successor to Dr. Hertzka's Hildegard Practice at Konstanz, West Germany in 1984. They have experimented with her remedies on a large scale and have found them effective. These remedies are worthy of experimentation in this country as well and give much for us to examine. They will contribute a new dimension to our understanding of herbal medicine. Hildegard's medicine will give us, moreover, a new understanding of the roots of our own Western herbal and natural-healing tradition. In addition, it will provide a new spiritual focus for our healing work that may help bring many of us back to our cultural origins.

DAVID FRAWLEY, O.M.D.
SANTA FE, NEW MEXICO
JULY 1987

David Frawley is co-author of The Yoga of Herbs *(1986)*
with Dr. Vasant Lad; and author of
The Creative Vision of the Early Upanishads *(1982);*
Beyond the Mind *(1984); and* Hymns from the
Golden Age *(1986).*

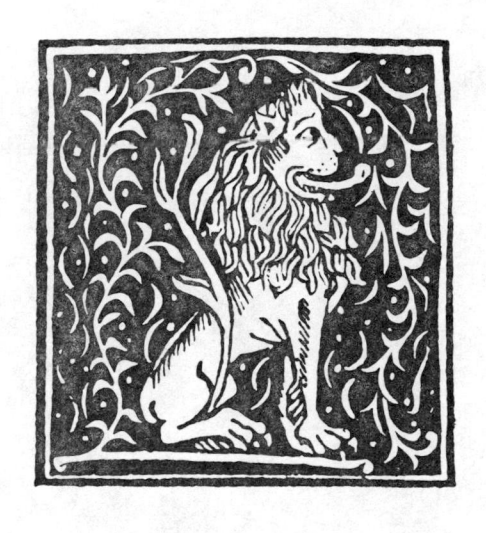

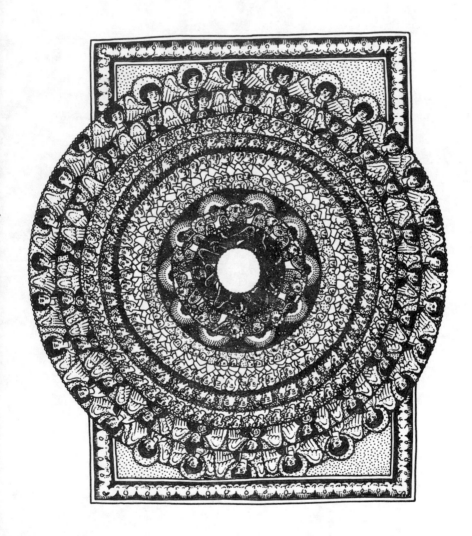

HILDEGARD'S MEDICINE
THE HEALING ART
OF THE FUTURE

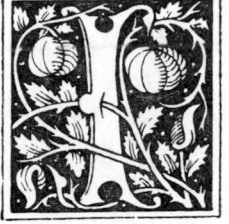 s there a need for a new sort of medical practice? That was the theme of a recent international doctor's conference, and the title of a book.

There is a great gap between the tremendous accomplishments in the treatment of accident victims and intensive care of the critically ill on the one hand, and on the other hand the helplessness with which we face the new chronic illnesses of our civilization, which are the cause of death for 80 percent of the population. In spite of great investments of money and effort in medical research, we still do not have a cure for heart attack, rheumatism, or cancer. And none will be found in the future, because the causes of these diseases cannot be discovered by the medicine of today with its natural science orientation, but rather by examining the incorrect way of life of the patient.

The best protection against these diseases can be found in proper diet (Hildegard diet), and in the elimination of spiritual risk-factors by means of a proper attitude towards life based on the strength and fullness of Christian faith, as it was revealed to Hildegard 800 years ago and recorded by her for our age.

This book is meant to be an important contribution towards bringing Hildegard medicine to the world. It is the result of decades of medical experience, and of scientific research and development in the field of Hildegard medicine. Over 500 remedies and methods of treatment have been tested by Dr. Hertzka and myself over the past forty years, and have proved to be a success for thousands of patients.

Hildegard is not just another collector of herbal remedies, which were so plentiful in the monastic medicine of her time. Rather, she obtained her knowledge through spiritual visions, which she herself experienced. In the last of her theology books, *Liber Divinorum Operum*, Hildegard of Bingen reveals the true author of the medical books which she wrote so many years ago on the Rupertsberg.

In all creation, trees, plants, animals, and gem stones, there are hidden secret powers which no person can know of unless they are revealed by God. (PL 893 C)

Hildegard was aware of her visionary gift and retained it until the end of her life. Thus, at age 70 she could say, "Everything I ever wrote came wholly from the source of my heavenly vision."(Pitra, 333; see page xxvi)

CONCERNING THE ORIGIN OF LIFE

The textbook of Hildegard's medicine has five chapters which correspond to the five senses. For the most part, the descriptions and themes of the textbook are identical with those of Hildegard's cosmic medicine as expounded in *Liber Divinorum Operum*, where they are presented again, but in an elaborated form. This is another proof of the visionary origin of her medicine.

In both books, Hildegard describes God as the source of all life. She speaks of the creation of angels, of the cosmos as the home for humanity, and of the sun, moon, and stars.

God was and is without beginning before the creation of the world. God was and is light and radiance and life. And God said, "Let there be light," and so were the light and the radiant angels created. (CC 1, 1)

The origin, sense, and goal of life are aptly expressed in the symbol of the radiant fiery angel. With his feet he treads upon Lucifer, the source of all evil, a monster of horrible features, venomous and black like a snake. (PL 743 B)

Lucifer is described as the origin of evil and sickness, which can be seen in the principle of atheism—the isolation and separation from God, the dissolution of the bond with life. "Health" and "healing" are related to the word "whole," which is the restoration of "one-ness" with God—the "at-one-ment" which brings health; and this is possible only with God's help. God is the whole life (*vita integra*):

All things burn through me . . . everything lives in my being and there is no death in it, since I am life itself. I am also the understanding. . .through which all creation is made. I breathe life into all things, so that nothing is mortal in its true nature. (PL 743 D)

Hildegard sees the cosmos as a world wheel, as a symbol for the infinite love which God shows humanity. The giant wheel is kept in motion by the power of the wind. In the center stands humanity with the four elements. Thus humankind is exposed to cosmic and atmospheric influences.

God created the world out of its elements to the glory of the divine name. God strengthened it with the wind, connected it to the stars and enlightened it by them, and filled it with all manner of creatures. God then surrounded and fulfilled humankind in the world with all things and gave them a tremendous power, so that all creation would support them in all things. The whole nature should serve them, so that they can live with it, because humankind cannot live or survive without nature. (PL 755 B)

In their original condition, people were placed by God in an upright position in the center of the cosmos, and they were wonderfully conceived and made.

Humans stand at the center of the cosmos, since they are of greater meaning than all other creatures which remain dependent on the world. Although they are small in stature, they are great in the power of their souls. Their heads are directed upwards and their feet stand on solid ground. Thus they are able to put the loftiest as well as the lowest things in motion. (PL 761 B)

The original world was in order. Humanity lived a kingly life with the support of all creation and without being oppressed by vices, sickness, or death.

O humankind, just look carefully at this [original] human! Heaven and earth and all created things were united in this original form and everything hidden within. (CC 2, 17 ff)

The world and all creation were made up of the four world-elements, the cosmic building blocks, which fill the world and all its creatures.

God also created the elements of the world. They are in humankind, who lives with them. They are called fire, air, water, and earth. These four basic elements are so closely connected and bound together that none can be separated from the others. Thus they hold so closely together that one can call them the basic building blocks of the cosmos. (CC 2, 37 ff)

The four world-elements have been well known in the field of medicine for many centuries. They are mentioned by physicians from Hippocrates to Paracelsus, and in even older sources. For Hildegard, the elements are the key to understanding the whole art of healing. The number four is not only significant in the construction of the cosmos, but also in the make-up and function of human beings, for example in the theory of the four humors, the four blood types, and the four temperaments and their characteristic variations in man and woman.

As has already been shown a number of times, just as the four elements hold the world together, they also form the structure for the human body. Their distribution and function in the whole human being are such that they constantly sustain the person, just as they are spread throughout all the rest of the world and have their effects. Fire, air, water, and earth are in humankind, and humans consist of them. From fire they have the warmth of their bodies, from air they have their breath, from water they have their blood and from earth their bodies [the materials of muscles and bones]. They can thank fire for their sight, air for their hearing, water for movement, and earth for their ability to walk. (CC 49, 29)

The four elements determine the constitution of the humors in a human being and thus the state of health. No one exists outside of this cosmic principle. Everything works together in this order, in balance and harmony, and thus a person remains healthy and alive.

When the elements fulfill their purpose correctly and orderly, so that warmth, dew, and rain come separately and in good measure and at the proper time, and maintain the earth and its fruits in health, and thus bring bountiful harvests and good health, then the world will prosper.

If they all come suddenly and at the same time, and not in their season, they would tear the earth apart and make it sick. Likewise, the elements maintain the health of person when they function in an orderly manner. As soon as they stray from this order, they make the person sick and cause death. As long as the flow of the humors in a person functions properly, and maintains warmth, moisture, blood, and flesh, then the person enjoys good health. But as soon as they flow all at once in excess and without caution, they create sickness and cause death. Warmth and moisture, as well as blood and flesh, were namely changed into the opposing phlegmata by Adam's fall into sin. (CC 49, 40)

Thus the original complete harmony in humankind was destroyed by the fall into sin. The various combinations of the fluids of the four world-elements resulted in a total of 24 basic illnesses.

However, a person who is saved (that is, healed) can achieve a still better state of health by means of proper Hildegard diagnosis and therapy.

WHAT IS A PROPER DIAGNOSIS?

According to Hildegard, there are not 6000 illnesses, as the modern medicine of today would have us believe. This diagnostic chaos is resolved in a clearly understandable basic principle in the medicine of Hildegard. In the process, one can look for guidance to the developmental history of a human being, just as modern science does. The three germinal layers from which the human body develops (ectoderm, mesoderm, and endoderm) form the basis for three large categories of illness:

Ectodermal Illnesses

The illnesses of the outer germinal layer have to do with the segmental structure of the body and the nervous system, that is, roughly within the skin. After all, the skin is a sense organ with many receptors which transmit a multitude of messages to the nervous system: sensations of temperature, pain, touch, and pressure. These illnesses affect the organs and are listed by Hildegard from head to toe: head, eyes, ears, teeth, heart, lungs, liver, spleen, stomach, kidneys, abdomen, sexual organs, gout of the big toe. These localized illnesses are inherited illnesses, with the typical weak points (Achilles heel) which a person brings into the world. They range from the scalp to the big toe. There is a specific treatment for each of these organs enumerated.

Mesodermal Illnesses

The mesomorphic illnesses of the middle germinal layer have to do with the connective tissue and the vessels. They are principally rheumatic and degenerative illnesses, colds, and the illnesses connected with elimination.

Endodermal Illnesses

The so-called serious internal illnesses, such as cancer, jaundice, dropsy, and intestinal illnesses, can be traced to the inner germinal layer, with a systematic listing of about forty types of illness. These internal ailments are largely connected with disturbances of the stomach and intestines, and can in part appear as eruptions of the skin. Likewise, skin ailments can be projected onto the intestines.

Nearly all illnesses can be classified according to this scheme of eighty general illnesses. Hildegard describes a thorough and reasonable therapy for each of them. A diagnosis according to the stature of a person, unique with Hildegard, is extremely important for a successful treatment. No complicated technical medical apparatus is necessary for the diagnosis, even though the Hildegard therapist is certainly free to use such an apparatus when it is felt that it may be of help.

Methods are even simpler in the more than 2000 remedies of *Physica*, in which ailing persons with good powers of observation can easily seek out the cure according to their own symptoms. If we had not had years of experience with Hildegard's healing art, we would not venture to make this book available to the public. Everything in it has been tested and proven in our practice. We must make one point clear: one can find relief from pain in many ways, including modern medicine. The spiritual equivalent of the illness must be addressed for a true healing. Every affliction has a meaning: What does God want to tell us with this illness?

A person who has been healed according to Hildegard's methods is thus healthier than before, something which cannot be said of most modern healing methods. Hildegard's healing art is preventative medicine. It is easier to prevent the illnesses of our modern civilization, such as heart and circulatory disease, than to treat them. The Hildegard diet and a proper way of life are more important than any cures or surgical treatments. So it is that there is hardly any place in our medicine for surgery. It is not unthinkable that a time will soon come when people will be amazed by the present effort to heal everything with surgery or wonder drugs such as cortisone and antibiotics.

The most important principle of treatment is the Hildegard diet. If we assume Hildegard to be right, then we must assume that diet is more important than any drug. The divine secrets of nourishment lie in a certain subtility, the name that Hildegard herself gave to her medical book. For Hildegard, subtility means those qualities which were hidden by God in the things of nature for the use of humanity, and which are known only to God, and by divine revelation. Only very few foods are 100-percent good for humans. Among them are spelt, chestnuts, and fennel.

For Hildegard, a healthy way of life is characterized by the general Christian attitude of moderation in all things—eating, sexuality, sleeping, and movement. Hildegard refers to this often in her textbook. She also tells of the influence wind, sun, the seasons, and places of cultivation can have upon diet and thus also upon human beings. She tells how the four elements (fire, air, water, and earth), and the quality of water and soil influence harvest and food.

With Hildegard, we are free of exaggeration. She prescribes neither extreme vegetarianism, nor a totally raw diet, nor is she a teetotaler. Wine and beer have a very meaningful dietetic function, both as medicine and as a beverage. What is important for Hildegard is the effect which a food or drink can have upon the disposition: whether it makes you happy or sad or has a negative psychic influence.

What cleanses our system of toxic substances? Humanity causes itself much affliction during the course of life through foolish habits such as overeating, from environmental contamination, or from the human violation of the harmony of creation, all of which lead to the production of bodily fluids which cause illnesses. For just such conditions, Hildegard has a great number of treatments which aid in the elimination of toxins and in cleansing the system through the skin by means of baths, saunas, packs, or rubbing in various preparations.

In addition, an "operation without a scalpel," in the form of a fasting cure, can play an important role as a universal means for finding a new attitude toward oneself. To achieve this purpose, a two-week Hildegard group cure is most often recommended. At the moment, there are so many books concerning fasting that we have included a chapter in this volume especially devoted to this theme.

Bloodletting is another age-old European therapy, which was already prescribed for all monasteries by Charlemagne. Every monastery was required to build a special house for the purpose of bloodletting. Today there are numerous scientific studies which show that this 1000-year-old technique of bloodletting, when properly applied, is capable of preventing heart attacks and strokes, since the patients prone to these afflictions have an extremely high blood viscosity and red corpuscle count.

The Hildegard practice of bloodletting "thins" the blood, makes it more fluid (lowers the hemostatic levels), and thus lessens the danger of thrombosis and stroke. This excellent treatment also eliminates toxins (black bile) in the blood which hinder healing, especially in patients with long histories of chronic illness. In addition, it stimulates the production of the body's own healing substances, such as cortisone. This treatment procedure so highly praised by Hildegard will be more widely followed in the future, for the prevention of illness and the healing of ailments already present.

Hildegard tells us how we can even predict the cause of an illness, and draw important conclusions, from the examination of the blood with is let. Hippocrates said, "One is to know the past (anamnesis), recognize the present (diagnosis) and predict the future (prognosis)." Hildegard even dedicated the fifth and last chapter of her textbook to the art of prognosis, an area much neglected in modern medicine.

In a similar manner, the cupping procedure is used in the treatment of many ailments, confirming the wonderful success

xxiv

which this treatment has enjoyed in China and Japan for thousands of years. But in this instance as well, Hildegard describes her own original procedure, which does not fit into the conventional Asiatic scheme.

Even the characteristic heat radiated by specific types of burning wood is used to therapeutic ends in the practice of Hildegard medicine. The use of elmwood fire, followed by kidney massage, in the treatment of kidney ailments and high blood pressure, has proved to be especially effective.

One can find many characteristic hints as to the further course of a person's health in the state of the eyes as windows to the soul, from the color of the skin, the sound of the voice, and the mood of the person. These phenomena have important consequences for the course of a treatment.

HILDEGARD'S MEDICAL BOOKS

In 1959, the Benedictine nuns Marianna Schrader and Adelgundis Führkötter, working together with historians and paleographers and with the support of the German society for research, proved the authenticity of the visionary trilogy mentioned below, and of more than 300 letters, compositions, and songs.

1. Book of Faith (*Scivias*)
2. Book of Life's Merits (*Liber Vitae Meritorum*)
3. Book of Divine Works (*Liber Divinorum Operum*)

Do the medical books belong to Hildegard's complete works?

The visionary phase involving medicine and natural science falls between the first and second works of Hildegard's trilogy. It was then that the medical book, *Subtilitates Diversarum Naturarum Creaturarum* (the explanation of the natural powers of the various creatures), was written. The work in its original form has not yet been found, but there are several copies of the following parts of the work.

1. *Liber Simplicis Medicinae* (the so-called book of healing methods or *Physica*): There are manuscripts of the first part of the work dating from the thirteenth to the fifteenth centuries located in Wolfenbüttel, Paris and Brussels, and an early printed copy

published by J. Scott in Strasbourg in 1533. The *Patrologia Latina* edition (Vol. 197, CPL, J.P. Migne, Paris, 1882) is based on this 1533 edition. A comparison of the various manuscripts shows that the integrity of the text has been carefully preserved (Heilmittel, Basel Hildegard Society, 1982).

2. *Liber Compositae Medicinae* (the book of composed medicine): The second part, with the title *Causae et Curae* (the causes and treatments of illness), was wonderfully preserved in a thirteenth century manuscript first discovered by Carl Jensen in 1859 in the Royal Library in Copenhagen. Cardinal J. Pitra published an excerpt in his *Analecta Sacra* (Vol. 8, Paris, 1881), and Karl Kaiser transcribed the complete text, printed with the title *Causae et Curae* in Berlin, 1903.

This book is important for the understanding of Hildegard's whole healing method and has come under careful critical scrutiny. The experts agree on the authenticity of the medical books ascribed to Hildegard; there has been no conclusive proof that they are spurious.

Hildegard's medical textbook is, in a sense, a summary of her last great theological medical book, *Liber Divinorum Operum*. It anticipates the later book, which elaborates the medical and cosmic interrelationship of humanity and the world in much greater detail.

FROM WHAT SOURCE
DID HILDEGARD TAKE HER MEDICINE?

The question of sources is very difficult in the case of Hildegard. As a prophet she refers only to the Bible. In a letter to Bernhard of Clairvaux dating from 1146 she says, "...I am an uneducated mortal and am in no way learned in things concerning the external world, but taught from within by means of my soul."(PL 189 C)

HILDEGARD HAS HER OWN LANGUAGE

Hildegard herself writes in Latin, but many ordinary Latin words have a special meaning when she uses them—for example *viriditas*, the greening power. The word does not occur in any other treatise on healing. Hildegard uses the word *viriditas* to refer to all living things, the energy of life which comes from

God, the power of youth and of sexuality, the power in seeds, the reproduction of cells, the power of regeneration, freshness, and creativity.

Weakness and loss of life-energy are the result of the tragedy of the loss of faith—the sin of allowing faith to dry out. A person who seems dried up has lost the power of creativity; the salvation from this desert, spiritual healing, comes as a gift of faith through Jesus Christ. For this reason, Hildegard refers to Mary as *viridissima virga*, the greenest virgin.

Another concept which Hildegard uses is that of black bile, *melanche*, which is the cause of melancholy. The medicine of Hildegard is based upon the principle that all internal processes in people can be traced back to biochemical origin. The substance which makes one sad and which plays a role in every serious illness, she calls black bile, which develops in humanity through the fall into sin.

With the fall into sin, the crystal-clear gallstone of Adam disintegrated into the black bile which is melanche proper, and into the gallic acids which are chemically related to the steroids, cholesterol, and sexual hormones. This melanche is always present in the blood, but at a higher level during illness. Many bodily and spiritual functions are influenced by the presence of these toxic substances which the body itself produces, and it is one of the greatest accomplishments of Hildegard medicine to eliminate these substances which cause illness and spiritual dysfunction. Antimelancholic remedies are based on this same principle of melanche neutralization. On the other hand, many improper life habits, such as the unaesthetic gulping of fast foods, can increase the levels of these depressive substances.

WHAT DOES HILDEGARD KNOW ABOUT THE PSYCHE OR SOUL?

Hildegard's medicine is a psychological or spiritual medicine. Hildegard not only wrote her own book on psychotherapy (*Liber Vitae Meritorum*), but also described common everyday aspects of psychological or spiritual functioning and how they affect the body. She compiled a list of 35 avoidable risk-factors, from nerve-wracking anger, and lust which ends in despair, to world weariness coming from a greed for possessions. Lack of faith is the cause of all evil, and faith increases the success of every cure.

Hildegard's healing art has one or more remedies for every ailment, but this does not mean that every person is curable by means of Hildegard's medicine. Even though most patients react positively to her remedies, Hildegard writes the following remarkable formulation in her textbook:

These remedies come from God and will either heal people or they must die, or God does not wish them to be healed. (CC 165, 21)

That is not a Solomon-like excuse for any possible failure. It has to do with only about one percent of her remedies, but they happen to be the most important cures. Certainly God wishes to heal everyone. Christ always healed those who pleaded for his aid.

The same is true of Hildegard, yet there are a certain few cases where God in divine wisdom realizes that curing the sick person will not help. It is obvious that Hildegard promotes Christian goals in the world and among humanity. We are reminded of the words of St. Augustine, "Omnia anima naturaliter christiana." The design of every soul is based on a Christian model. It is in this sense that all of Hildegard's books are to be understood, including her medical books.

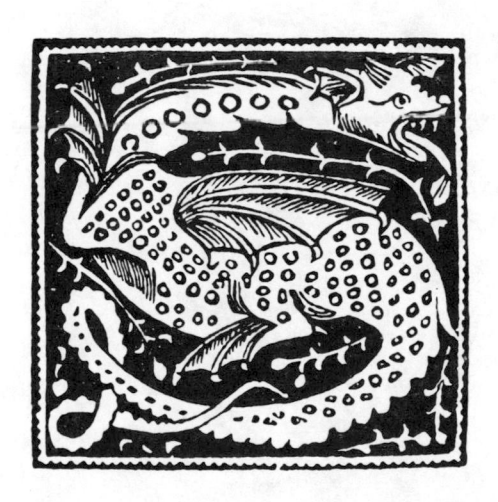

HILDEGARD'S
MEDICINE

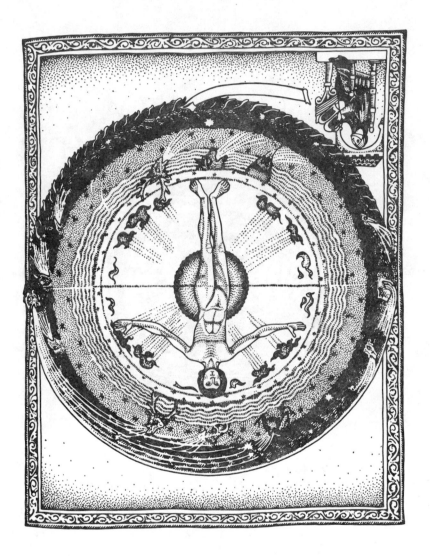

Chapter One

EYES

THE WINDOWS TO THE SOUL

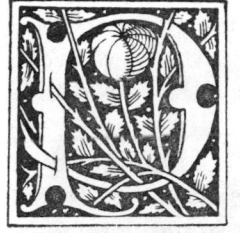

owerful is the expression of the soul in the eyes of this person, when the eyes are clear and shining, because the soul is energetically living in the body, so that it can accomplish many works within. For the eyes of a person are the windows to the soul. (CC 220, 6)

Bright eyes are signs of life. If someone is physically healthy, he or she has clear and sparkling eyes.

Dull eyes are signs of death!

Whoever, on the other hand, does not have shining eyes, no matter what color, even though the person is healthy, bears the sign of death. Also, when the eyes are dim like a cloud which is so dense on the surface that behind it the transparent cloud cannot be seen, then such a person will become sick soon and death will follow. In the look of the eyes of a person like that the soul, namely, is not powerful, because it will hardly create anything there and in a manner of speaking sits there covered by clouds, like a man who is considering and is in doubt when he should leave his home and go out of his house. (CC 220, 11)

In modern medical terminology, the eye is a complex and delicate structure. The tough outer layer or sclera is visible as the white of the eye. A circle of muscle (ciliary body) supports and controls the lens. The ciliary skin secretes aqueous humor, a watery liquid, which fills the anterior and posterior chambers between cornea and iris. The iris is the colored portion of the eye and regulates the amount of light by adjusting the size of its central opening, the pupil. The visual image is focused on the retina.

It is interesting to compare the above with Hildegard's version:

The pupil of the eye has a similarity with the sun; the black or grey coloring around the pupil compares to the moon, and the white, lying outermost, is like the clouds. The eye is made up of fire and water. Through fire it is held together and strengthened, so it can exist; the water, on the other hand, makes seeing possible. If blood spreads on the surface of the eye, it will suppress the vision of the eye, because it dries out the water which bestows vision to the eye. On the other hand, if blood is excessively reduced there, water, which enables the eye to see, will not have enough strength; it should carry strengths in blood like a column. For that reason the eyes of old people become weak in vision, because they are losing their strength and the water with the blood is decreasing. That is why young people can see more sharply than old, because in their vessels the right proportion exists between blood and water. (CC 92, 7)

Hildegard describes five types of eyes according to their color: blue-grey eyes, fiery eyes, eyes of diverse colors, turbulent eyes, and black eyes. Blue-eyed persons are thoughtless, rash, unwise, mischievous, daring, willful, lazy, and disorderly, but they bring everything to a good ending.

A person who has blue eyes like water gets them mainly from the air. That is why they are weaker than other eyes, because air shifts often as a result of the diverse movement produced through warmth, cold, and humidity, and such eyes are easily harmed by bad, soft, and moist air as well as by fog. For just like these affect the purity of air adversely, they also harm eyes acquired from the air. (CC 92, 24)

Fennel (*Foeniculum vulgare*), one of Hildegard's favorite plants, is the universal remedy for blue eyes. Even the side effects of modern-day air pollution, very harmful for air-sensitive blue eyes, can be eliminated by fennel.

If someone has blue eyes, with which she somehow sees poorly and feels pain, she should take fennel or fennel seeds when the pain is fresh, pulverize them, press the juice from them, and take the dew which is found on grass blades standing upright, add a little fine wheat flour, and knead this into a little cake. This she should place over her eyes for the night, tie it in place, and she will feel better. The mild warmth of fennel, tempered by the dew and the strength of the flour, removes these pains. Grey eyes are the airy kind, and therefore dew is added to this mild medicine. (CC 170, 14)

Fiery eyes have a ring around the iris and can be either blue or brown. Those with fiery eyes are clever, hot-tempered, energetic, and keen-minded, and their eyes are healthy.

Whoever has fiery eyes, comparable to the dark cloud next to the sun, received them naturally from the warm south wind. They are healthy, because they originate from the warmth of the fire.(CC 92, 32)

Fiery eyes are irritated by dust, smoke and other types of air pollution. In Hildegard's words:

Dust, however, and bad smell injures them, because their brightness disregards dust and their purity neglects the unfamiliar smell.

(CC 92, 35)

Fiery eyes suffering from all forms of eye ailments are restored to health with rose-violet-fennel wine. The recipe calls for six milliliters (ml.) of violet tincture, twelve ml. rose tincture and four ml. fennel tincture added to enough wine to make fifty ml. medicine.

Rub this eye water around the eyes before going to bed, being careful not to hurt them accidentally through the strong effect. (CC 170, 27)

The third type of eyes have a color mixed from blue or grey—spotted eyes, eyes with diverse colors in them. Persons with such eyes are up one minute, down the next, fickle and inconstant; but honesty and respectability characterize individuals with number-three-type eyes.

Whoever has eyes like the cloud in which the rainbow is shining received them from the air of the various air currents, which are neither constantly dry nor moist. They are weak, because they come into being from the unstable, changing air; and, because they do not originate from fire, they have an obscure vision by warm air, whereas by pure rainy air they can see clearly; this is because they are more of a watery than fiery kind. Everything, especially bright light from the sun, the moon, lights and from the splendor of precious stones or metals or something else, is harmful for such eyes, because they come from the air with its changing currents. (CC 93, 1)

Eyes "like a cloud" are the poor television eyes extremely sensitive to light. Prolonged eye stress from watching long movies, or excessive TV or reading, irritate and pain these eyes,

5

sometimes causing blurring, double vision or seeing flashing lights or floating spots. In persons over fifty, the lens of the eye may cloud, a possible cause of cataracts. Modern medicine relates the cataract to an impaired glucose-utilization due to a loss of enzymes in the lens. The decreased enzyme activity can be stimulated by Hildegard's zinc wine, thereby regenerating vision. Zinc wine can be a prophylactic and therapeutic remedy for cataracts and early glaucoma, as well as a very helpful eye medication for pink eye (conjunctivitis). Even itchy, irritated eyes with excessive tears due to an allergy such as hay fever, or irritation from wind, dust, smoke or air pollution, are soothed with zinc wine. For all forms of acute or chronic conjunctivitis:

The person should take zinc oxide and put it in pure white wine. At night when this person goes to bed, he or she should take the zinc oxide out again and wet the eyelashes with the wine, being careful not to touch the eyes inside and thereby hurt them through the bite of the zinc oxide so that they become even weaker in vision. Zinc oxide has just as much warmth as cold and, tempered with the warmth of the wine, gets rid of the harmful juices which make the eyes sick. (CC 171, 6)

The eyes of the fourth type are green and rare. Hildegard describes them as cloudy or similar to a storm cloud.

About turbulent eyes: Whoever has eyes which are like a storm cloud, neither completely turbulent, but rather somewhat greenish-blue, received them from the dark dampness of the earth that brings forth diverse, useless herbs and even earthworms. They are gentle and have prominent red flesh, which originates from slime. They are irritated by neither moist air nor dust, by bad smell nor bright light from any object, ... although they sometimes suffer from certain other ailments.

(CC 93, 12)

People with green eyes are good craftsmen and very good at learning a new trade. Other characteristics include instability and cunningness.

Whoever has eyes like a dark cloud, more greenish in color—and suffers weakness of vision and pain—should pulverize fennel herbs (leaves) in the summertime, or fennel seeds in the winter, and carefully mix them with egg white; when he gets ready to sleep he should put it on his eyes. The gentle warmth of the fennel diminished by the cold of the egg white will reduce the weakness of vision and pain in such eyes.

(CC 171, 19)

The sharpest eyes are type number five: "black eyes," or brown eyes, as we would call them.

A person who has very black or dark turbulent eyes, like a cloud, received them primarily from the earth. They are stronger and see more keenly than any other eyes and keep the keenness for a long time, because they come from the energy of the earth. But they are easily injured by the moisture of the earth and the wetness of rain and swamps, just like the earth is also poisoned by harmful moisture and the great wetness of rains and swamps. (CC 93, 25)

Brown-eyed people are clever and accept good advice, but they often feel cramped. If their eyes hurt or trouble them, the rue tincture compress will bring relief.

Take rue juice, and twice as much pure liquid honey, and add a little pure good wine. Lay a piece of wheat bread in this mixture, and then tie it on the eyes with the bread overnight. (CC 171, 33-35)

Impaired eye vision can be a result of acute glaucoma, a serious disorder caused by increased pressure due to excess fluid inside the eye. Hypertension of the eye, or glaucoma, deteriorates vision, so that it may eventually lead to permanent blindness. Even without symptoms, like blurred vision and pain in or around the eye, everyone over forty should have a periodic eye examination and glaucoma test. The earlier the treatment, the greater the chance for success. Hildegard suggests very simply:

When blood and water decrease the eyes of a person too much because of age or sickness, this person should go to a green grassy garden yard and look at it for as long as the eyes are wet like from crying, because the green of the grass takes away whatever cloudiness was in the eyes and makes them clear and bright. One can also go to a river or pour fresh water in a bowl and, leaning over, catch the wetness of this water with the eyes. This wetness re-activates the water in the eyes, which was drying up, and makes them clear. One can also take a linen cloth, dip it in pure cold water, and lay it over the temples and eyes, tying it, being careful not to touch the eyes on the inside, . . . (CC 169, 30)

Grapevine drippings is a universal eye remedy from Hildegard and is excellent for a beginning cataract. A progressive painless loss of vision in middle-aged or older people is characteristic of both cataracts and glaucoma and can be helped by

7

grapevine drippings.

Anyone with blurry and cloudy eyes [beginning cataract] should lubricate the eyelids often [daily] with the grape drops, which run out of the vine after cutting, and allow a little to run into the eye. This will clear the eyes without a doubt. (PL 1244 D)

Another good rejuvenating procedure for treatment of early stages of cataract is apple blossom extract mixed in equal parts with grapevine drops. Irritated, itching eyes with too many tears, as typically found in pinkeye, allergic syndrome (hay fever), acute conjunctivitis caused by bacteria, or irritation from wind, dust, smoke and air pollution, can be relieved by Hildegard's apple blossom/grape drops:

A person, old or young, disturbed from any kind of clouding of the eyes, should take apple blossoms and leaves in the springtime before fruit appears. When the leaves first come out, they are tender and healthy like a maiden, before she bears children. Squeeze the juice out of its blossoms and leaves and add it to equal parts of grapevine drippings, mix and fill it in a bottle. At night, before going to sleep, moisten the eyelids and the eyes [with your fingertip], so that nothing penetrates the eyes. Then moisten the leaves with the grape drops and put them on the eyes [as a compress] overnight. If you do this often [daily], the opacity will disappear and you will be able to see more clearly. (PL 1215 D)

Sometimes a degenerative opacity of the lens occurs as a result of an inflammation, senility, effects of X-ray, trauma, or diabetes, as well as ingestion of certain toxic substances or drugs. Vision lost through cataracts can be corrected by surgery, but deterioration due to glaucoma mistakenly diagnosed as a cataract may lead to permanent blindness.

Gold topaz is one of the best remedies for vision loss:

Whoever has a [progressive] loss of vision should lay a topaz three days and nights in pure wine. Moisten your eyes at night before you go to sleep with the moist topaz, so that the liquid also runs in the eyes. This wine can be used for five days, after removing the topaz. Moisten the eyes every night with the topaz dipped in wine. After five days renew the wine, following the above procedure. This clears the eyes like the best eye medicine. (PL 1255 C)

Impaired vision caused by hormone disturbances from the thyroid, which darken and blur vision, may benefit from a rock crystal:

Put the rock crystal in the sun and put the warm crystal on your eyes, if they are blurry. The rock crystal eliminates the malicious fluids [unshed tears, as in glaucoma with its big inner pressure] and the person will regain vision, because its natural art originates from water.
(PL 1263 D)

Another precious stone, the blue sapphire, relieves the pain of pinkeye (conjunctivitis):

Whoever has painful eyes, red and inflamed, or impaired vision, should place a sapphire in the mouth before breakfast and moisten it with saliva. Then this person should take the saliva with the fingertips and moisten the eyes, so that the inner eye is touched by the sapphire. The eyes will be healed and very clear.   (PL 1253 C)

Painful eyes can be associated with an acute glaucoma attack. Always call your physician, because untreated glaucoma can result in permanent blindness.

Our eyes are a mirror reflecting the mood of the soul. By looking deeply into the eyes and reading their body language, simple things like a smile, or tears in the eyes, can identify grief or joy. But eyes, according to Hildegard, are also related to the first pair of virtues and vices: love of heavenly things and love of the world. As found in 1 John 2:15, "Do not love the world or the things in the world. If anyone loves the world, love for the Father is not in him. For all that is in the world, the lust of the flesh and the lust of the eyes and the pride of life, is not of the Father but is of the world."

Our eyes can be fooled by a materialistic or wrong world-outlook, so that the invisible world (the inner world) is not a reality at all. Psalms 135:16b, "They have eyes, but they see not," or Psalms 119:18, "Open my eyes, that I may behold wondrous things out of thy law." Seeing is believing, if we only know how to see.

"Lighten my eyes," pleads the Psalmist (Psalms 13:3b), "lest I sleep the sleep of death." Physical death is not meant here, but rather spiritual death, which we find in our modern world more than ever before. So let us be alive, seeing with open, sparkling, uplifted eyes and joining in this prayer of praise: "To thee I lift up my eyes, O thou who art enthroned in the heavens! Behold, as the eyes of servants look to the hand of their master, as the eyes of a maid to the hand of her mistress, so our eyes look to the Lord our God, till mercy be had upon us." (Psalms 123:1-2)

Chapter Two

EARS
L I V E R
M E T A B O L I S M &
H E A R I N G

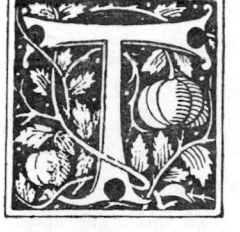 *he two ears are like two wings, which lead all the voices and tones in and out, just like wings carry the birds into the air.*

Every sickness has not only a cause. It has a meaning and purpose. Sometimes it teaches us to control our stomach more carefully. In June, when strawberries are ripe, earaches, tonsil infections, sore throats, appendicitis, and rashes increase dramatically. Hildegard writes:

The fruits, namely the strawberries, adversely affect persons who eat them [change the blood chemistry], and they are not good to eat for either the healthy or the sick, because they grow close to the earth and because they even grow in foul air. (PL 1194 A)

Similar problems occur, by the way, when eating peaches.

Most people will not condemn the strawberry or peach, at least not immediately. But whoever suffers from any of the above-mentioned maladies should restrain his or her palate and learn to give up these pleasures early in life, so as to be spared many other sicknesses.

In early spring, when the grapevines are trimmed, the sap can be collected as an effective ointment for earache.

Collect the sap from the trimmings in a very clean bottle between early morning and noon [not later, otherwise the sap will spoil], and store it in a dark room. (PL 1244 D)

The sap itself is not only an effective ear remedy, but a fantastic eye medication, even in various cases of pinkeye. Moisten your eyelid with the sap once or twice daily and you will have improved vision. From this grapevine dripping, fill a small medicine bottle nine-tenths full and then add olive oil the other one-tenth, and shake well before use. *(Guttae vitis oleosae [rosatum]*H).

This remedy treats earache, even pain of middle-ear infections, as well as headache in cases of neuralgia where there is pain in and around the ear. Dip your finger in and rub the fluid all around your ear thoroughly, not inside the ear like other eardrops. It provides quick, effective relief, and prevents early outbreak of middle-ear infection. In cases of acute middle-ear infection, it relieves the pain; however if fever is present, see your doctor. This oily grapevine preparation is so helpful, no home or travelling first-aid kit should be without it.

Another tested remedy for temporary deafness requires the use of an oblong stone, the jasper. Hildegard describes the procedure:

If persons are deaf in one ear, they should breathe on a jasper so that it becomes warm and moist from their breath. Then they should place the stone immediately into their ear and close up the rest of the ear canal with soft cotton, so that the warmth of the stone is transferred to the ear. In this way they will recover their hearing. (PL 1257 A)

For this purpose, the jasper stone is cut and polished in an olive shape, like a small bean, and then fastened to a little chain so that the stone cannot slip too deeply into the ear canal. Likewise, a cone-shaped jasper may be used which only partially fits into the ear canal and cannot slide any deeper.

A powder mixed from four ingredients treats deafness caused by catarrh and infection of the middle ear (galangal-aloe powder):

Hildegard writes:

Take galangal [catarrh root], and one-third that quantity aloe, and twice that quantity oregano, and also some peach leaves. Make a powder out of these and use it daily after eating as well as on an empty stomach. (PL 1135 A)

Patients using this powder take one or two pinches to "spice" their last bite of a meal or with their food.

The ear plays an important part in body metabolism resulting from an interplay with the liver. Hildegard sees a direct relationship between that which the ear hears and the metabolism of the liver. The sounds of loud disco music cannot only hurt the ear but can also perforate the liver like Swiss cheese. Good music, on the other hand, normalizes the low metabolism of depressed persons and fills them with joy.

The ear is, according to Hildegard, a very important center controlling health and disease:

Whenever the blood vessels come in contact with body fluids which have been shocked in such a manner, then they also reach the vessels of the ears and now and then affect the hearing capability, because often a person earns health or sickness with hearing; similarly, the person is overjoyed with happiness, but with misfortune falls into deep sorrow.

(LDO III, vision)

The familiar concept of ancient doctors—healing with music—arose from the same ideas. Hildegard herself composed over 77 chants and a musical drama, "Ordo Virtutem." Now that we finally know that mental disturbances (distress, resentment, misery) can be healed with music, it also would be worthwhile to investigate how the metabolism of the liver is normalized. (See Chapter Nine.)

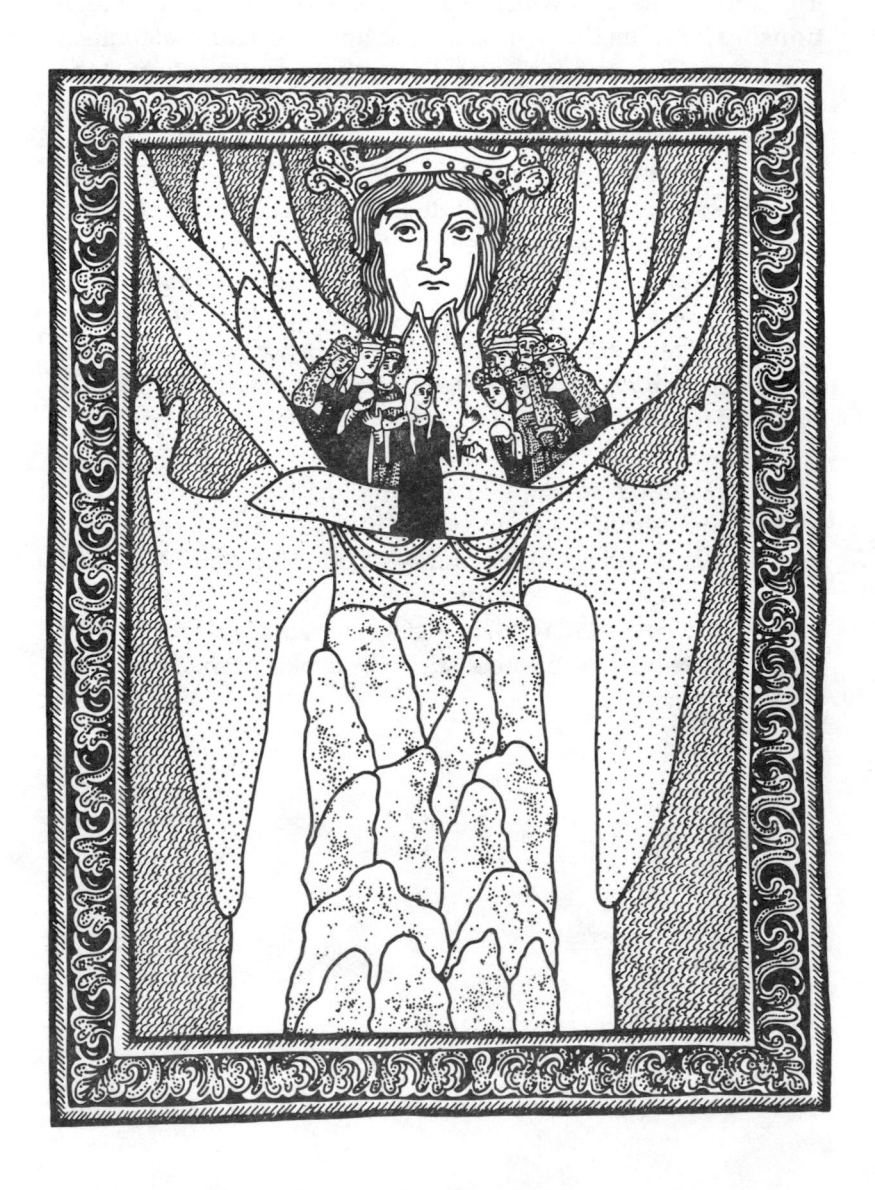

Chapter Three

TEETH

A BEAUTIFUL SMILE

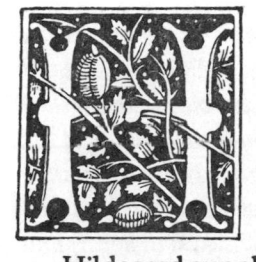ildegard's method for preventing cavities and treating periodontal disease is an absolutely dependable method from today's scientific viewpoint. How could she know and provide such effective remedies for the present if they were not inspired by the wisdom of God?

Hildegard supplies us with a simple and effective procedure for every day, called cold-water hardening. Those who desire strong, healthy teeth, should rinse the mouth with fresh, clean water immediately upon arising in the morning (CC 173, 33). Hold the water in your mouth until the sticky film on your teeth dissolves. Brush your teeth often and repeatedly with cold clean water. The build-up of film will not increase and your teeth will be strong and healthy.

Cold-water hardening is a most effective and powerful tool for strong teeth. Get into the habit of brushing immediately upon arising, with cold, fresh water (spring or well water is best without toothpaste, flouride, chloride, or any other adulterant). Cold water dissolves mucous plaque, cleans stains and discoloration from teeth, and leaves a fresh taste in the mouth. Get your family acquainted with this practice early on, because warm-water brushing softens teeth.

For everyday tooth care, Hildegard suggests the grapevine ash tonic:

If your gums are decayed, add [pulverized] grapevine ash, still warm, to a good wine. Brush your teeth often, and after dinner daily. Your teeth and gums will become strengthened. For those who have healthy teeth, maintain this procedure for a vital and healthy smile.

(PL 1244 B)

Take a mouthful of grape-ash wine and brush teeth and gums with it, using a soft bristled brush. Don't rinse, just spit it out. It is an effective treatment for bleeding gums and periodontosis, and it promotes bright, shiny teeth. Sore gums will regenerate themselves with new cells and hold the teeth firmly again.

Hildegard gives us a precise, almost pathological explanation for the onset of dental caries (i.e. tooth decay).

The very finest vessels surround the thin skin, or membrane, in which the brain lies, and extend to the gums and teeth themselves. If they are filled with bad, terrible smelling and rotten blood, and if they are impurified through the scum which occurs by the cleansing of the brain, then they carry the rotten matter with its pain from the brain to the gums and into the teeth themselves. In this way the meat that surrounds the teeth of such a person, and even the cheek, will swell, and then the person will have pain in his gums. Whenever a person does not clean his teeth frequently by rinsing with water, a slime will grow occasionally in the gums and accumulate. In this way the gums become sick and sometimes worms appear in the teeth from the old slime, and the gums swell and the person has pain. (CC 94, 17)

In order to restore the health and growth of new cells, one can apply the toothache wine. It is effective in cleaning and removing decayed waste material and irritants. The wine is extremely helpful in treating severe tooth and gum pain, and should always be used when one has irritation after drilling or root filling.

Whoever suffers from toxic blood [infections], or through discharges from the brain to the teeth, should take equal parts of vermouth [one to two tablespoons] and vervain [Verbena officinalis], and cook them in a clean container with pure natural wine. Strain the wine and drink it after adding some sugar. The cooked herbs, still warm, should be placed on the jaw, where the toothache is, and tied with a cloth before going to sleep. This the person should do until healed. The wine tempered with the above-mentioned herbs, then drunk, cleans the little vessels extend-

ing from the cerebral membrane to the gums from the inside. The herbs placed on the jaw placate the toothache from the outside, because the warmth of vermouth with the warmth of vervain and that of the wine calms down the toothache. (CC 173, 14)

The herbs are available in teabags ready to use as a compress. The toothache wine is also effective in eliminating the so-called "foci" caused by bacteria, viruses, and particularly silver amalgam fillings. These fillings are extremely poisonous, because they continually release small amounts of mercury that destroy the immune system.

Hildegard provides us with remedies against dental caries and periodontal decay that result from our daily intake of today's devitalized, demineralized foods, such as sugar, candy, and refined white flour.

When a worm is eating the teeth of a person, he or she should take equal amounts of powdered aloe [Aloe vera] and myrrh. Heat this mixture over the glowing coals of beechwood in a pottery receptacle with a narrow opening. Let the rising smoke get to the painful teeth through slightly opened lips by way of a straw. The teeth themselves, however, must be tightly closed, so that not too much smoke enters the throat. Do this two to three times a day for five days and you will be healed.

(CC 174, 5)

According to Hildegard, the heat of the aloe and myrrh, invigorated by the burning coals, will kill the bacteria. Who will be the ingenious technician to construct a cavity "smoke gun" for the teeth of Hildegard fans?

In order to treat and prevent periodontal disease and gum inflammation, take the *viriditas* (life energy) of fresh green leaves: "Take garden lettuce, or, when not available, freshcut leaves, and add a bit of chervil. Chop thoroughly. Add some wine and chew this for fifteen to twenty minutes." (PL 1165 B) This method is consistent with scientific evidence that chlorophyll has effective, remedial qualities.

Calcium deficiency is another cause of periodontal disease. How could Hildegard know that we need salmon bone powder (*Salmonis pulverata*) as a basic cure for calcium deficiencies? When your teeth decay and weaken, pulverize salmon fish bone to a powder (one teaspoon) and add a pinch of salt. Before bed, brush with this mixture, but do not rinse. This will cleanse your gums, remove yellow stains, eliminate plaque, heal and strengthen your teeth. (PL 1274 D)

Chapter Four

COLDS & FLU
& THE ENGLISH GERANIUM

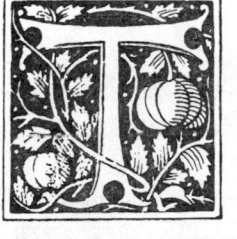

he common cold starts with a loud "a-choo!" "God bless you!"
Why do we sneeze? Hildegard has a new and interesting answer:
Whenever the blood in the vessels is not awake and lively, but rather just lies there as if it were sleeping, and also when the body liquids don't move fast enough, but are lazy and slow, the soul notices this and causes the body to tremble through sneezing and in this way wakes up the blood and juices of the person so that they return to their correct behavior. If water is not moved through storms and floods, it will foul. In the same way a person, who would not sneeze or blow the nose to clean it, will foul from the inside!   (CC 133, 9)

Surprisingly enough, Hildegard has a helpful selection of remedies to treat and prevent the common cold. The most universal of all these remedies is flu powder, which has powdered English geranium as its main ingredient. For six common symptoms this unique flu powder is a versatile and effective remedy. (See Chapter Six.)

1. Runny nose:
smell, don't sniff, flu powder several times a day after blowing your nose.
2. Headache caused by flu or by weather sensitivity:
2—3 pinches of flu powder with salt on bread.
3. Sore throat, hoarseness:
1 teaspoon flu powder cooked for 2 minutes with a glass of wine; drink while warm.

4. Coughing:
1 teaspoon flu powder mixed in a pancake (spelt or whole wheat flour, water, salt, no egg) together with cinnamon, and apple sauce several times a day.

5. Stomach flu:
1 teaspoon flu powder after meals.(PL 1188 B)

6. Heart pain during and after flu:
in order to avoid further heart damage caused by toxins from flu virus infection, take 2-3 pinches of flu powder every day on salad or bread, or lick it out of your hand. (PL 1188 A)

7. Preventive medicine:
½ teaspoon flu powder in salad or soup during a flu epidemic or season for colds; it is almost 100% effective.

When a cold or flu is at its worst, fever joins the other symptoms. Like other old herbalists, Hildegard praises the rootstock of the imperial masterwort (*Radix Imperatoria ostruthium*) for its effectiveness against all fever conditions:

Masterwort is warm and reduces fever. Whoever has any kind of fever should take masterwort [rootstock], chop it a little [one teaspoon] pour half a glass of wine over it, leave it in the wine over night, and the next morning add wine to it again and then drink it before breakfast for three to five days. (PL 1193 A)

Repeat this procedure every evening using fresh masterwort; in severe cases, for five days. Strain the juice and take a teaspoonful several times a day before eating.

Another very simple but effective fever remedy, excellent for children, is galangal-raspberry water. Two tablets of galangal (one-third teaspoon galangal powder) are crushed and stirred into a glass of raspberry juice (made from raspberry syrup and water). This pleasant-tasting medicine should be sipped often throughout the day. Don't forget to stir it each time!

Whenever a sickness is accompanied by fever, it is advisable to remain in bed in a warm but not overheated room. Moisten the air with steam from a kettle of hot water, or a humidifier. Drink plenty of herbal tea (fennel, sage) and freshly squeezed orange and lemon juice. Stop eating and follow the diet for the sick, stages one to three. (See Chapter Eight.)

Hildegard differentiates very precisely between colds with coughing and colds with a sore throat. Colds with simple coughing require the horehound tonic (*Marrubium vulgare compositum*):

Those who cough should take fennel and dill in equal parts, add one-third of a part of horehound and boil the herbs in wine, strain through a linen cloth, drink, and the cough will disappear. (PL 1143 A)

Patients who suffer from a sore throat with rough and raw feelings should drink mullein tonic (*Verbascum thapsus compositum*):

Those who have a sore throat and hoarseness with pain in their chest cook mullein and fennel in equal parts in pure wine, strain it through a linen cloth, and drink often [daily], and their lost voice will return again.   (PL 1180 B)

The combination of both tonics is an excellent treatment for all cases of runny nose, coughing, and hoarseness; it is called *spezies grippales compositum* (mullein, fennel, dill, and horehound) and is prepared as above. The blockage of the nose by a thick and opaque discharge, together with pressure and pain in the sinuses (sinusitis), is a result of assorted noxious fluids (*diversis humores*) according to Hildegard. These fluids originate in our food and drink. Some foods, especially dairy products such as creamy milk, cheese, and ice cream, cause noxious slime which blocks the nose. Grownups, who often lack lactase, find dairy products hard to digest. Cheese can be made more readily digestible by spicing with cumin.

Hildegard herself explains the runny nose in a wonderful way:

Although the human brain is mostly healthy and pure, sometimes disturbances of the air and the other elements rise up to the brain and pull various humors [fluids] back and forth to the brain, causing a foggy smoke to appear in the passages of the nose and throat, so that a harmful slime collects there like the smoke of foggy water. This slime draws the diseased parts of the weak fluids together, so that they are painfully secreted out of nose and throat; similarly, ulcers break open when they are ripe and the slime in them drains; and no food can be cooked without ridding itself of impurities through the cleansing foam. In the same manner the soul works in the human body, when all the body fluids in the eyes, ears, nose, mouth, and digestive tract—each in their own

21

way—are cooked through the fire of the soul, like a food is cooked over the fire, until it brings up foam. (CC 134, 19)

Fuming herbs (*herbulae fumantes*) mixed from the tender tips of fennel and dill are an excellent help for severe runny nose. The sick person takes a clean earthenware flower pot and heats it on the stove until it is very warm, but not too hot. Then one teaspoon of fuming herbs is sprinkled on the hot earthenware so that it smokes. Inhale the rising fumes in mouth and nose, if necessary through the use of a funnel placed upside down over the flower pot to concentrate the fumes. When the inhalation is finished, toast a piece of bread and eat it with the roasted herbs. Do this for three to five evenings (also during the day) and the worst runny nose will get better.(PL 1157 B)

Hay fever is tormenting more and more people, especially children, due to weak resistance and an overload of environmental poisons. But there is a help to overcome symptoms such as a stuffed swollen nose with clear watery discharge, itchy eyes and repeated sneezing. The jasper nose olive will help to clear the nose and provide a better ventilation:

Whoever has a strong thick discharge should take a jasper and breath on it so that it gets moist and warm from the warm breath. Then the jasper is put in the nostril and covered with the hand, so that the warmness of the stone rises up to the brain. Now the phlegm will dissolve much more easily and the person will get well again.(PL 1257 A)

Another excellent treatment for hay fever is inhaling the fumes from smoking yew-tree wood (*Taxus baccata*). Cut a small dry piece of wood into shavings and heat them in a clean flower pot on the stove. Inhale this smoke through nose and mouth daily for at least a week and the hay fever will be relieved.

Whoever has an ailment in nose and chest caused by virulent fluids should inhale the smoke from yew wood in nose and mouth and the virulent fluids will dissolve gently and comfortably and disappear without harm from the body. (PL 1238 C)

Asthma, together with migraine, is very difficult to heal. A severe attack of asthma, in which the patient is fighting for breath and becomes pale and clammy with a blue tinge to the tongue, is an emergency, and admission to the hospital is essential. In order to help the lungs, the patient should drink goat's milk. It is easy to digest and high in vitamins A, B, and D. The fat particles are smaller than those of cow's milk. Goat's milk is naturally homogenized and doesn't separate.

Whoever has an unhealthy lung shall drink enough goat's milk and be cured.					(PL 1325 B)

Everyone with lung disorders, especially asthmatics, should drink one pint of goat's milk a day.

Chronic bronchitis with wheezing, especially if accompanied by breathlessness, or painful breathing, or if accompanied by coughing up of grey or greenish-yellow phlegm, needs a cure with hart's tongue fern tonic. It is a very unique treatment for a patient with an impaired liver function and intestinal disorder resulting from malfunction of the hormones.

Hart's tongue fern [Scolopendrium vulgare] is warm and helps painful liver, lung, and intestinal ailments. Take hart's tongue fern and cook in strong wine, add pure honey, boil up again, add long pepper [Piper Longum] and twice as much cinnamon, and boil a third time; strain through a linen cloth to make a clear tonic, and drink often [daily] before and after meals. It benefits the liver, cleanses the lung, and heals the aching intestines.					(PL 1142 A/B)

This very curative treatment has been helpful in cases of impaired function of endocrine glands, such as menstrual disorders, cystitis, gallbladder inflammation and insulin starvation due to diabetes.

Like the healing soups in Chinese medicine, horehound cream soup, eaten three or four times, will heal chronic infections of tonsils, throat, larynx, and sinuses. Take one to two tablespoons, or for sore throat and sinusitis a handful of cut horehound herbs, and cook in one cup of water. Strain the horehound water and add two cups of (white) wine. Cook one cup of this mixture with two to three tablespoons of cream for a bowl of soup.

Drink often daily and the throat will be healed.		(PL 1143 A)

As a result of heart disease, old people sometimes develop emphysema, suffering shortness of breath without any physical exertion. They have the feeling that they cannot get enough air; breathing is painful and they have a dry cough. There is no curative treatment available in modern medicine. Only Hildegard's

23

lungwort wine may help relieve the symptoms and finally increase the oxygen intake.

Whoever has an inflated lung, so that he or she coughs and breathes with difficulty, should cook lungwort [Pulmonaria officinalis] in wine and drink it often on an empty stomach, and he or she will be healed.

(PL 1141 D)

Patients with these same symptoms, but without coughing, should prepare lungwort tea (with water) and drink before and after meals three times a day until cured.

The tea removes bad breath and harmful phlegm causing difficulties in breathing and pain in the lung. (CC 175 B)

The leaves of common columbine flowers (*Aquilegia vulgaris*) provide another simple remedy. They should be chewed raw, several times a day for several weeks, by everyone with swollen glands or adenoid problems. A six-year-old boy, who could no longer hear well, came to my office this summer. His adenoids were blocking the eustachian tube to such degree that an immediate operation was indicated. With a lymph drainage treatment and regular columbine drops, the boy gradually improved, so that an operation was no longer necessary. By September he had regained his normal hearing and could begin school.

Craving and curiosity for new and unfamiliar foods and drinks may be the origin of the runny nose. The body, in its wisdom, tries to eliminate the resulting toxins as liquids through the nose. This cleansing procedure is just as important as digestion and elimination, and should never be blocked by nosedrops or other means.

In the light of Hildegard's cause-and-effect relationship, it may be craving for entertainment (joculatrix = third vice) which causes a stuffed or runny nose. The return to health requires not only moderation in food and drink (modesty = third virtue), but also simplicity of life style.

Add the simple almond, eating five to six nuts a day, to an uncomplicated life style and we have Hildegard's cold preventative. As mentioned in the Old Testament, the almond tree with its manifold fruits is a symbol not only for Mary but also for *viriditas.* When Moses went into the tent of the testimony on the

24

morning after all twelve leaders had deposited their rods inside, he found Aaron's rod had sprouted, put forth buds, produced blossoms, and bore ripe almonds (Numbers 17:8). And of these almonds Hildegard writes:

The bark, the leaves, and the sap are not good as remedies, because all its energy is concentrated in the fruit. But whoever has an empty brain, a face of bad color, and headaches should often eat the inside pits of this fruit, and it will fill the brain and give him the right color. But whoever is lung sick and has a defective liver should eat these nuts often, either raw or cooked, and they will bring energy to the lungs, because they don't steam or dry the person in any way, but rather strengthen him or her. (PL 1225 C/D)

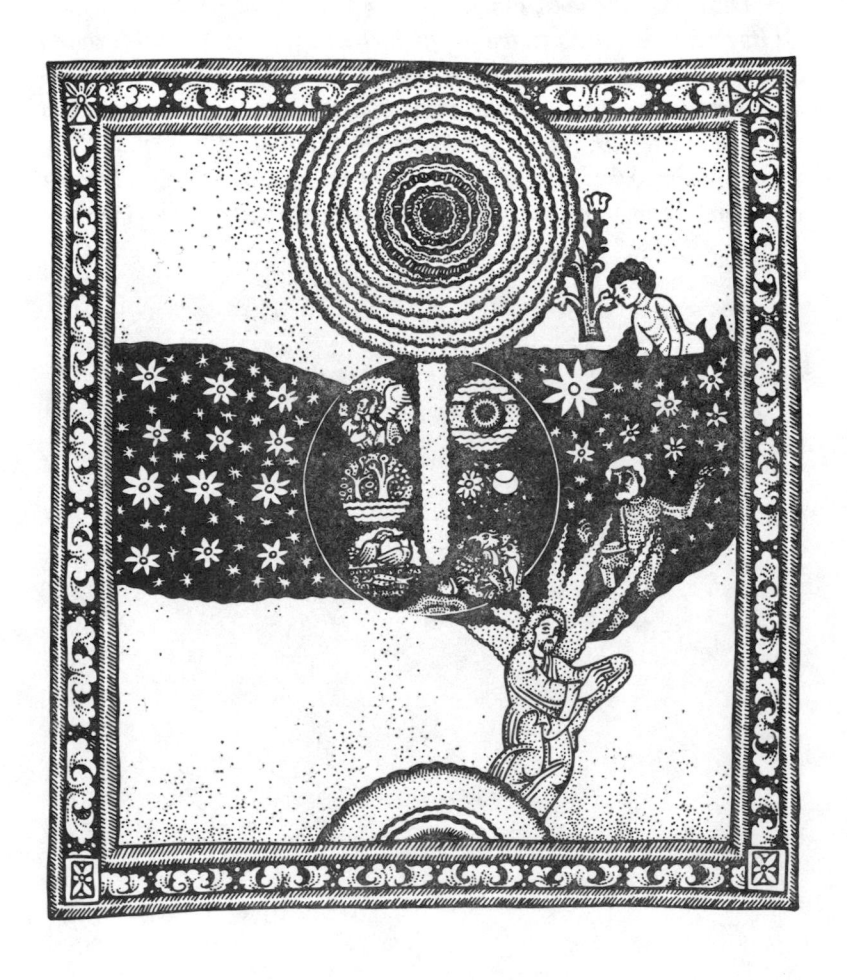

Chapter Five

SKIN

CUTS, BITES & BURNS

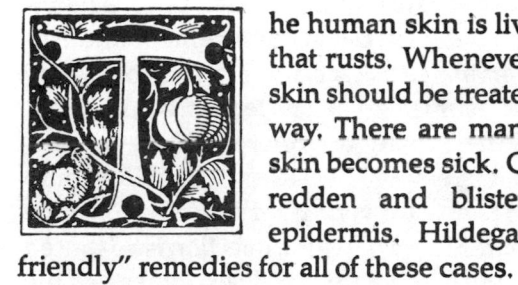he human skin is living; it is not like iron that rusts. Whenever the skin is sick, the skin should be treated in a "skin-friendly" way. There are many ways in which the skin becomes sick. Cuts may infect, burns redden and blister, bites plague the epidermis. Hildegard has many "skin-friendly" remedies for all of these cases.

Healing through the skin plays a very prominent role in the Hildegardian system of treatment. Many Hildegard remedies operate through the skin, such as rubbings, baths, warming, sauna, cupping, etc. Skin problems are the least treated, and internal diseases the most treated, with these methods.

Rash, a common skin problem, is described by Hildegard:

When bad humours afflict an individual with a rash on his entire body, one should wait awhile until the abscesses mature and the humours are discharged. When the skin between the abscesses turns red and begins to dry out, a suitable salve should be applied without delay. In this way, the skin will not become more painful through the infection and will not relapse into sepsis. (CC 154, 33)

Probably the best of Hildegard's skin remedies is the violet salve, which is effective against scar tissue:

Take violets, press their juice, and strain it. Weigh olive oil to one-third the weight of the violet juice, and take goat's fat exactly the same weight as the juice. Let these three ingredients simmer in a new pot and it will become a salve. (CC 204, 25)

Hildegard never concerns herself with the causes of illness through germs, because it is completely impossible to kill all the bacteria, viruses, and bugs which cause infections of the skin. The human skin plays a major role as a defense wall against infection. Mostly the innate self-healing power of the body is sufficient to fight infection, if the correct remedies are used to stimulate it. To some extent it depends upon the aggressiveness of the infecting germs, and certainly upon our intelligence, not to turn a small pus pocket, which would clear up on its own, into a large abscess by provoking it with scratching or squeezing.

An infection is always the result of a preceding wound, and it is important to know what to do when there is a serious festering or inflammation. Do not wait; begin the treatment immediately with European vervain (*Verbena officinalis*) as soon as any infection becomes troublesome and begins to form a pus pocket anywhere on the skin, in the skin, or under the skin.

In advanced cases it is usually necessary for the doctor to lance the abscess. This is an old, very good procedure, which allows the pus to flow out. But whether the infection is advanced or not, a vervain compress will stop the development of the infection. It makes the infected area more resistant, so that bacteria can no longer spread.

The vervain treatment must be done properly. First, the infected area has to be covered with a clean, ironed piece of linen, and then the boiled herb, not the water, should be placed on the linen while still warm. One tablespoon of ground vervain can be put into a single sack of muslin, which can be easily made by sewing a seam along the edges. The sack is then boiled in water and, after pressing out some of the water, the sack with the warm vervain is placed on the linen cloth which covers the abscess. As soon as it is dry, the process should be repeated. (PL 1190 B)

In this way, many simple infections can be nipped in the bud, and more advanced ones arrested. After lancing the abscess, if that is necessary, the treatment promotes rapid wound healing. Once a wound has become infected and persists for more than three days, it is wise to consult your physician for diagnosis and treatment. Only the physician can decide if the patient should be given additional antibiotic treatment. If the vervain method is applied early enough, a natural wound-healing results from the body's own curative power.

ABSCESS AS A RESULT OF
A SKIN DISEASE OF SCROFULOUS NATURE

The lymphatic glands along the neck may become visible and sensitive, even though there is no pain anywhere else. There are often a number of them in a row, like a string of pearls. They mostly do not hurt but become a matter of concern for mothers, because they are stubbornly present for weeks or months. Sometimes they form actual bundles and can become so big that they burst. That used to be called "scrofula" or "pig's neck", because pigs characteristically have a heavy deposit on their necks. Skin abscesses of a scrofulous nature are most often a result of a tuberculous infection of lymphatic glands. Mostly children are afflicted with such "neck glands".

We are not talking about those knots or lymphatic glands on the neck, which can be felt in the region of the jaw and ear, and which become painful or sensitive in cases of tonsilitis, diptheria, scarlet fever, or any inflammation in the area of the head, ears, teeth, etc. They have to do with some pocket of infection, will disappear with that infection, and need no special treatment. Usually, the physician takes notice of them only as a symptom of a basic illness, such as a sore throat, earache, toothache, etc.

In the case of scrofulous disease, good results can be obtained from a very simple remedy: raw columbine (*Aquilegia vulgaris*) leaves should be chewed several times a day for several weeks (PL 1184 B). Where these lovely garden flowers grow there is no problem. They seed themselves and show up every year, almost like weeds. At least that is true of the most common varieties.

Probably, the wild meadow columbines have the same healing powers, but I would not say that they must definitely be wild. On the contrary, careful cultivation and domestication by people always ennobles wild varieties. Hildegard says that to a certain degree the effort invested improves the heritage.

The washed leaves may be dipped in honey or chopped up

and mixed with apple sauce, quince compote or similar neutral, i.e. unharmful, flavor bases, and even finicky children will enjoy eating them. If dried columbines (preferably leaves) from the druggist are used, one should proceed as follows: Mix fifty grams of powdered columbines with twenty to thirty grams of columbine tincture (columbine juice in alcohol) and give the patient two teaspoonfuls daily mixed with apple sauce. If the results are not satisfactory after several weeks or months, there is no choice but to turn to the original recipe and use fresh columbine leaves.

BURNS

The linseed compress is a simple and safe method of treatment for all ordinary household burns, which often take place in the kitchen. Even third-degree burns with charred skin and scabs can be brought under control by a linseed compress. Burns due to radiation, including X-rays, will likewise show good results with a linseed compress.

The advantages of the linseed compress are so many, it is hard to know which one to mention first. Every burn is accompanied by pain and "heat," both of which can be instantly relieved using this remedy. An immediate application of the linseed bandage prevents infection. In a beautiful and safe way, an uncomplicated wound-healing follows quickly, without too much unsightly scar tissue.

Whoever is burned anywhere on the body should cook linseeds vigorously in water, soak a sterile [ironed] linen cloth in this water, place it warm on the burned spot, and it will draw out the burn. (PL 1202 D)

About three teaspoons of whole linseeds (*Linum usitatissimum*) should be boiled in two cups of water (one-half liter). Cook the seeds until the water turns slimy, like jelly. (Careful, it foams heavily!) Then strain, as only the liquid is used. For the compress one must take linen cloth, because apparently the fiber also has a healing effect on burns. This corresponds exactly with a modern idea—that it is important what sort of dressing material (contact substance) is used. The linen cloth soaked with linseed water is placed *warm* on the burn and replaced as soon as it begins to dry out or become unpleasantly cold.

30

When the "heat" which has caused the actual burn damage has been drawn out and there is a normal skin wound left, the linseed-water bandage should be removed and the usual burn salves used. After the skin is restored, there remains only a normal wound like other skin wounds.

INSECT BITES

It is an irritating phenomenon of the summer to be plagued by insect bites at home and on vacation. Mosquitoes, flies, horse flies, bees and wasps are waiting—especially in August—at every turn and have robbed more than a few of the joy of fresh air and sunshine. If these beasts have spotted you as a possible victim, you will do well to get acquainted with this cheap and abundant remedy. Since rubbing and scratching will not get rid of the itch of an insect bite, you are better off following this tried and tested remedy.

Plantain is warm and dry. . . . if a spider or another worm touches or stings a person, then this person should immediately rub the spot with plantain juice and he or she will be better. (PL 1169 C)

The broad leaf of the well-known plantain weed is found growing along the edges of most fields and even disfiguring our lawns. The thin, pointed leaf of the ribgrass (English plantain) is equally well suited for this treatment. Press the juice from clean leaves, washing them first, if necessary, and put it on the bite. If there is strong itching or swelling, rub the juice in several times and put the crushed leaves on the wound. It is a surprise to experience such quick and thorough relief.

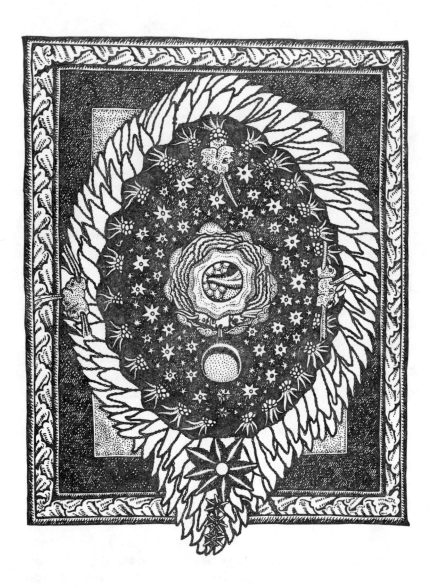

Chapter Six

HEART

GALANGAL &
JASPER

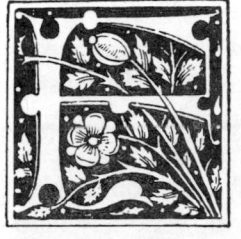
or out of the abundance of the heart the mouth speaks". (Matthew 12:34)
Jesus said, "Why do you think evil in your hearts?" (Mark 9:4)
"...and does not doubt in his heart,..." (Mark 11:23)
"But Mary kept all these things, pondering them in her heart." (Luke 2:19)

What do these four biblical passages have in common? Hildegard helps us with the answer. She points out that it is not the brain that "thinks," but rather the heart, and that the heart can be called "the thought factory." Thoughts represent labeled messenger-molecules which are formed, stamped, and pressed in the heart. They circulate in the blood until they reach their destination. There the thoughts adhere and cause reactions in the liver, the kidneys, and in many other places. What a contrast this description of heart disease is to the following.

According to the Framingham study of the National Heart Institute, cardiovascular disease is caused by malnutrition and five severe risk factors:

1. High blood pressure.
2. High cholesterol blood level, causing arteriosclerosis.
3. Clotting of the blood.
4. Smoking, coffee, alcohol, drug addiction.
5. Obesity.

Conventional medicine treats cardiovascular disease essentially by attempting to eliminate these five factors, without focusing on the underlying causes. Hildegard looks beyond the surface and obvious symptoms, and describes the 35 vices that conceive these problems. She also provides 35 heart remedies that correlate with these underlying vices. The heart acts as headquarters, where the impact of words, thoughts, and emotions leave their signals.

In the course of anyone's life, the time will come when the heart begins to hurt. Everybody should always bear in mind that not every heart pain is necessarily a sickness or an indication of old age. It depends on you, or your family doctor, whether you let yourself be classified as a heart patient, or if you consider the pain a warning from your heart to change your life style. If one tries to get rid of the discomfort immediately with a strong medicine, one will probably ignore the deeper intention of God and become a heart patient for life. For some people, heart pain can be a warning to reflect on their emotions and beliefs, or to completely change their way of living. Others may be encouraged to throw away cigarettes, not to take things (life) too seriously, or to make peace with their neighbor (enemy) and to learn to control their anger and temper; or perhaps just to thank God that they are still alive. The pain is a precursor and is meant to remind you that God could claim you tomorrow unless you repent your ways today. Hildegard's 35 heart remedies can be seen as a humanistic healing approach, because they acknowledge the real causes.

Whenever you feel pain in your heart, spleen, or side, parsley-honeywine is a great help. Think about your life style. Throw away your cigarettes. Do not work so hard at night. Perhaps you require more exercise, hiking, or walking. Do not overeat. One who is oversensitive to the remarks of others is constantly irritating the heart. Concentrating on materialistic rather than spiritual matters, such as money-making or money-losing, creates turmoil instead of peace. Confront anger and other negative thought patterns. Release your negative energy and develop a spiritual attitude. And take the parsley-honeywine!

Hildegard's parsley-honeywine is a delicious and effective remedy and it is easy to make. This ideal combination of heart medicine and heart tonic does relieve pains in the heart, spleen, and side.

Take eight to ten parsley leaves with stems. Boil in one quart of natural red or white wine with two tablespoons wine vinegar for five minutes. Add three-quarters cup honey (one-third cup or less for diabetics) and heat up again for five minutes. Skim off the foam, strain, and rebottle the wine. (PL 1159 A)

Take one to three tablespoons daily and all gripping, shooting heart pain, caused by weather or excitement, will disappear. You don't have to be afraid—heart wine can never harm you. Not only the initial light heart pain disappears, but even severe heart pain caused by chronic rheumatic disease or by heart insufficiency can be healed. Parsley-honeywine is valuable in cases of rehabilitation after heart attacks, too. It does not matter whether you use red or white wine, but it should be a natural wine, without additives.

The parsley-honeywine is one of the best tonics, well known to Hildegard patients and even to Americans. During my first workshop in Valparaiso, Indiana, at the Art Barn, I was happy to hear of one lady's experience with the wine during the past two years. She had suffered a heart attack and had had continuous heart pain and significant alterations in her electrocardiogram. For two years her heart pain has been gone and her electrocardiogram has returned to a normal pattern. She no longer requires the heart wine, but faithfully takes one tablespoon daily as a preventative measure.

Through overeating, or from a diet saturated with fat or raw foods, the heart muscle can also be damaged. In addition to heart pain, such excesses can cause fatigue, mood changes, possible loss of weight, and sometimes loss of consciousness. Hildegard writes:

If the stomach is irritated through different harmful foods and the bladder weakened through miscellaneous detrimental drinks, then they both will bring bad juices to the intestines and send a foul smoke to the spleen. The spleen will swell and become sore, and through its swelling and soreness create heart pain and cause slime to appear around the heart. But the heart is still strong and offers resistance to the heart pain. If, however, the previously mentioned juices increase in the intestines and spleen of the person and also bring the heart much trouble, then they will turn back to the black bile and mix together. Irritated through this the black bile, together with the other juices, will rise angrily toward the heart with a black, foul smoke and tire it through numerous afflictions occurring suddenly. That is why such persons are sad and grouchy and eat and drink so little that they lose weight and sometimes can hardly stand upright. (CC 95, 13)

The heart cure will strengthen the heart organ. According to the experience of many heart patients, the heart cure should be taken as follows for the best results: Take three heart pills (see below) three times daily for three weeks (in the first week after eating, in the second and third week between meals). Drink one liqueur glass of heart juice (see below) three times a day right after taking the pills. In cases of additional heart or chest pain, also take one to three pinches of heart powder (see below) on a dry piece of bread, especially after eating or excitement. Fear of heart attacks causes heart attacks. Bread with heart powder will get rid of this fear and create peace, relaxation and a certain sense of security. This three-week heart cure, comprised of heart pills, heart juice, and heart powder, is a basic curative treatment to fortify the heart.

To prepare heart pills, Hildegard writes:

Take galangal and pellitory [Anacyclus pyrethrum] in equal parts, add [one-quarter of the above amount] white pepper and mix this with beanmeal [fava bean (Farine fabae)]. Add juice from fenugreek without water, wine, or any other liquid. Form small pills, dry them in the sunshine, and this will lessen heart pain. (CC 174, 21)

To prepare heart juice:

Take licorice, five times as much fennel seeds, sugar with the same weight as the licorice, and a little honey. Prepare a drink out of these ingredients [by adding water], and drink for heart pain. (CC 175, 1)

In addition to this, prepare heart powder as follows:

Take white pepper, one-third cumin, and add as much fenugreek as cumin. Powder this, put on bread, and eat it for heart pain. (CC 175, 7)

Flu is a tricky illness for those who have not taken enough time to completely overcome it. Toxins caused by bacteria or viruses are responsible for heart damage after flu. This damage can be prevented with Hildegard's flu powder.

During and after flu:

Take herb Robert [Geranium robertianum—we found Gera-

nium anglicum *more potent], a little less pellitory* [Anacyclus pyrethrum] *and nutmeg and mix the powder. Those who have heart pain should eat this powder [two to three pinches] with or without bread, because it is the best powder for the health of your heart.*

(PL 1188 A)

At the onset of flu, take two to three pinches of flu powder every day for four weeks.

One of the most exciting discoveries of Hildegard medicine is galangal (*Alpinia galanga*), a very potent, quick-acting heart pain reliever. This friend and helper protects against angina pectoris, heart attacks, and gall bladder attacks caused by gastro-cardial pressure after heavy meals. Galangal is just as effective as nitroglycerin without any undesirable side effects. In no other medicinal folk book on Earth can you find a reference to galangal as a heart pain reliever. Only Hildegard describes the use of galangal in her *Physica*:

Whoever has heart pain and is weak in the heart should instantly eat enough galangal, and he or she will be well again. (PL 1134 A)

If there would be a drug to wake up the dead, then galangal would be the first choice. Related to the ginger family, it is the hottest spice on Earth, and an important ingredient in the curries of Oriental cuisine. Like a friend from Sri Lanka who always took her box of curry spices with her wherever she travelled, it is best for everyone to have galangal available in every situation: in the pocket, in the glove compartment, and at the bedside.

The German FDA (BGA in Berlin) has recently proved galangal safe and effective. The active mechanism of galangal is based on its active substances: bioflavonoids, essential oils, and hot-tasting ingredients which in their entirety have spasmolytic, carminative (cleansing), and pain-killing properties. In any cases of chest or heart pain, fainting, dizziness, fatigue, or collapse, place one galangal tablet (one or two-tenths of a gram) immediately under the tongue and rest a while. Its spasmolytic action opens the cramped blood vessels, may lower blood pressure, and increases the oxygen supply through better circulation. It relieves the symptoms without being habit-forming.

A delicious galangal recipe is galangal honey (five to thirty percent) as a daily breakfast spread. The pleasant habit of eating

37

galangal honey stops "sticky blood cells" from adhesion and helps prevent blood clots (thrombosis), a major cause of heart attacks. One example of many is the patient who had a heart cramp nine years ago and has had no recurrence simply through enjoying galangal honey.

Those with extreme heart weakness and a fear of impending death may benefit from Hildegard's yellow gentian soup.

Those who have such severe heart pain that their heart feels like it is barely hanging by a thread, take yellow gentian [Gentiana lutea, two to three pinches daily] in a [spelt flour] soup and their heart will be strengthened. (PL 1142 B/C)

This soup, taken daily for a week, is extremely helpful for the anxious patient who has a long history of heart disorder.

The gemstone jasper is the pacemaker for the suffering heart, especially in cases of critical conditions with arrhythmic episodes, heart pain, fluttering, or violent rheumatic attacks. Press the cool jasper firmly over your heart, directly on the skin, and take it away after a few minutes when it is hot. After it cools, put it on again and repeat the process three to five times, or as often as necessary.

When the body fluids violently attack and cause a storm called "gout" [a sort of rheumatic fever attack] in one's heart, in the loins, or anywhere else in the body, place a jasper on that spot and hold it there until it becomes warm—and the gout will vanish, beacause the good warmth and the good power will heal and calm down those bad warm and bad cold fluids. (PL 1257 B)

The jasper cooling is a unique remedy, since "gout" in Hildegard medicine means a variety of rheumatic sicknesses with symptoms like heart pain, acute arrhythmas, cerebral and renal complication, and sciatic pains. In all these cases the jasper stone helps and heals.

The emerald possesses a similar healing power to the parsley-honeywine. With its greenness (*viriditas*) the emerald changes "debility and infirmity" back into health.

Those whose heart, stomach, or side hurts should have an emerald by them, so that the flesh of the body becomes warm and they will get better. (PL 1249 B)

The emerald can be fastened with a bandage either right on the heart or in the navel, and it will strengthen dried-up life energy with its green fire. On a chain or in a ring, the emerald can be a great help for all congenitally handicapped persons for whom no other help is available.

Food for the heart, as in Hildegard's diet, is the most effective method to prevent heart disease (see Chapter Eight). In accordance with modern medicine, Hildegard's diet cuts back on foods high in fats and cholesterol to avoid the development of arteriosclerosis, and recommends that salt should be eaten in moderation to prevent hypertension. The following should be avoided:

1. saturated fats:
animal fats, dairy fats, cream, ice cream, solid vegetable fats, coconut, palm oil, and fried foods.
2. cholesterol:
egg yolks, skin from poultry, ground hamburger, shellfish and carp, shrimp, caviar, kidney, brain, and tongue.
3. salt:
no more than 1 level tablespoon (3 grams) a day; don't forget that cheese, dressing, bread, etc. also contain salt.

Limit alcohol to one serving a day (no hard liquor). One serving equals two ounces of dry wine or five ounces of beer. Increase polyunsaturated fat through seafood (all fresh fish)—cod, haddock, flounder, shad, swordfish, salmon, halibut, trout, pike, and sole; and fats of plant origin—liquid safflower, soybean, or corn oil (cold pressed).

New scientific research is discovering what Hildegard knew 800 years ago—that eating the right kinds of foods may lower the risk of heart disease. By changing the chemistry of your blood, the right kind of fish may retard the development of arteriosclerosis, a killer that strangles the heart's arteries. Researchers have studied the seafood-eating habits of the Eskimos of Greenland and the Japanese, and have found that their seafood diet protects them from heart disease. Salmon is especially rich in fatty acids, which have the ability to lower cholesterol levels in the blood and prevent heart attacks.

ARTERIOSCLEROSIS
Arteriosclerosis is characteristically silent for decades, until it is finally recognized in middle-aged or older persons. Probably the first symptom noticed is a general tiredness during the day, causing a gradual loss of energy and concentration. Later on, hardening of the arteries causes forgetfulness, confusion, and personality change, with depression and irritability. This most important disease of the blood vessels is the forerunner of angina pectoris, heart attacks, impaired circulation, and strokes. In its advanced stage, arteriosclerosis causes severe malfunction in all organs, especially in the liver, lung, and kidney.

Hildegard describes arteriosclerosis as a chain reaction beginning with an impaired kidney function and an overproduction of black bile (*melanche*), causing melancholy. This phenomenon is called the "loins sickness" by Hildegard and pinpoints the kidney as the main cause of premature aging. The toxic waste products, which can no longer be properly eliminated, accumulate in the body and settle as deposits in tissues and vessels. A film darkens the vision of the eye, clogged arteries weaken the heart and lung, and digestion is poor, blocking the intake of essential nutrients.

Hildegard's spring tonic prevents arteriosclerosis and cleanses the body of waste products:

When vermouth is young and fresh, press the juice and strain it; and then boil wine with a little honey and pour this juice into the wine, so that the taste of the juice predominates over that of the honeywine, and drink it before breakfast from May to October every other day. It suppresses the loins sickness and melancholy in you; it clears the eyes, strengthens the heart, and prevents the lungs from becoming sick; and it warms the stomach and cleans the intestines, providing a good digestion. (PL 1173 B)

Memory oil is a successful treatment for persons becoming silly, forgetful, or senseless:

Persons who are forgetful against their wishes should take stinging nettles and pulverize them, add olive oil, and rub their chest and temples energetically when going to bed; this they should repeat and their forgetfullness will decrease. The pungent warmth of the stinging nettles

and the warmth of the olive oil stimulate the constricted vessels of the chest and temples, which sleep a little by waking consciousness.
(CC 195, 13)

The chestnut, like spelt and fennel, is totally healthful and relieves all infirmities in people, as Hildegard says. Chestnuts are an extremely helpful brain food for people who develop arteriosclerosis, particularly sclerosis of the brain, including Alzheimer's disease, with symptoms such as loss of memory, dizziness, arteriosclerotic headache, etc.

A person whose brain is empty and dry, and who is therefore weak in the head, should cook chestnuts in water [twenty to thirty minutes] and eat them often [daily]. The brain will improve and be filled up, and the nerves will be strengthened, and in this way the head affliction will vanish. (PL 1227 A)

Besides valuable protein, chestnuts contain an abundance of bioflavonoids and vitamins A, B, and C, together with neurotransmitters (gaba) for the proper nerve function. Chestnuts supply a wealth of high value carbohydrates (22-34 percent) as energy for the brain. It is very important to know that chestnuts can be recommended for diabetics, as they do not contain glucose or fructose. The fruits contain 45-58 percent starch, providing 210 calories in 100 grams (approximately three ounce serving). Out of the wisdom of God, Hildegard wrote 800 years ago that the chestnut is an ideal brain and nerve food, a friend and helper of all persons over forty. Even today scientists have not fully understood, or are only beginning to understand, that proper food is good health.

41

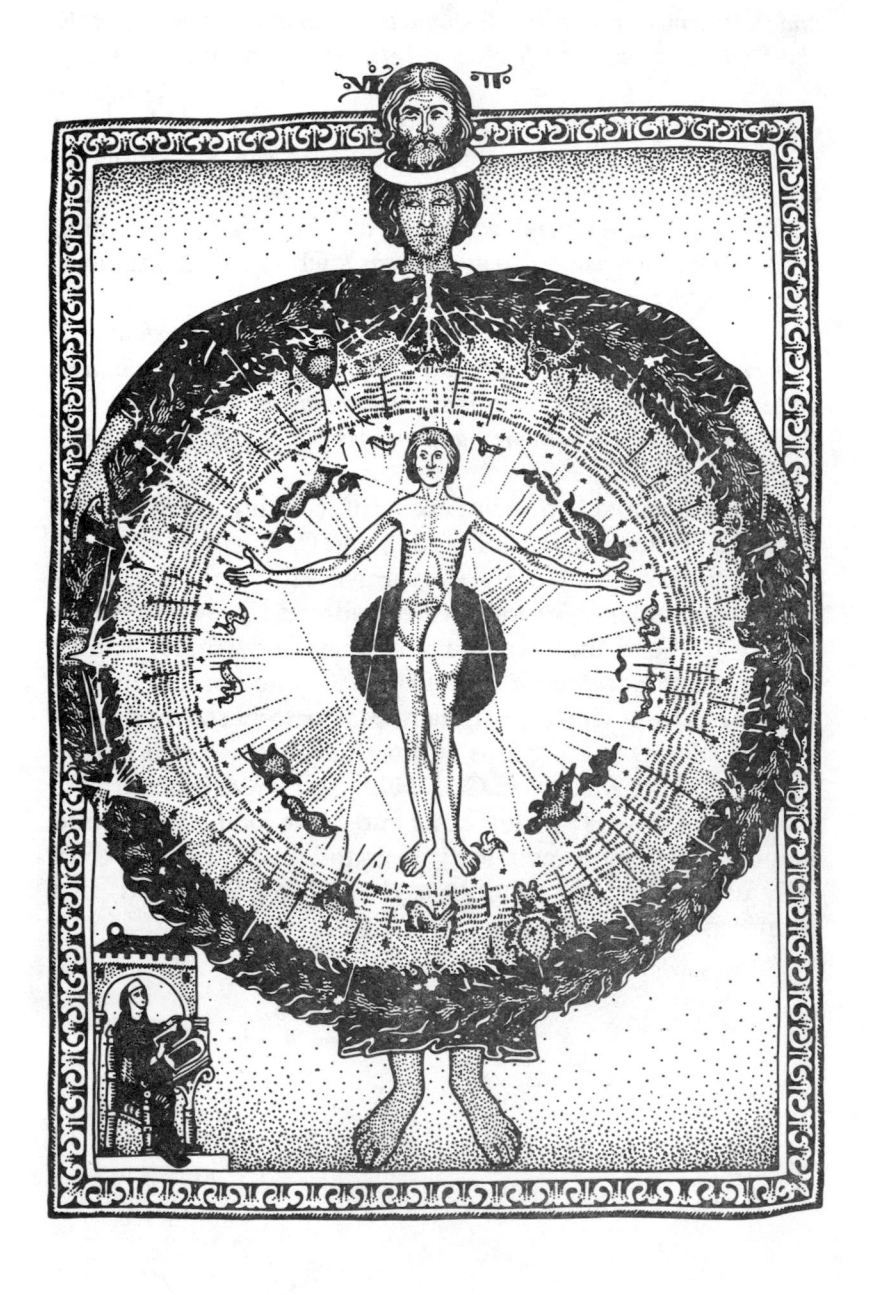

Chapter Seven

DIGESTION

& THE
WONDER FOOD
SPELT

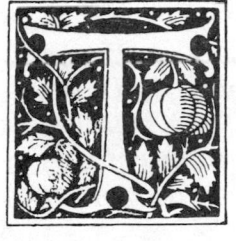he stomach has been created in the human body *for the purpose of absorbing and digesting all foods. It is tough and somewhat wrinkled on the inside, so that it can retain the food for digestion and not let it slip away too quickly to the stool. In the same way, the bricklayer roughens the stone, so that it will take on the mortar and hold it tight, and it will not run apart and fall on the earth.* (CC 99, 5)

It is universally accepted today that a proper digestion is a powerful key to health, happiness, and long life. A poor digestion is the main cause of modern complaints like nervousness, fatigue, chronic aches and pains, overweight, high blood pressure, and the loss of resistance to disease. Aging and disease begin when the normal regeneration process slows down.

Body restoration dries up, like Hildegard says, due to poor digestion and ineffective assimilation. Each cell needs an optimal supply of nutritional substances such as proteins, carbohydrates, fats, vitamins, and minerals, as well as fresh air and water. Tissues also require constant cleansing through the elimination of dead and dying cells, toxins, and waste materials.

Hildegard gives us very precise directions for an optimal digestion. She describes the reason for a good bowel function and moderate eating habits. Following her instructions gives one the best available knowledge of how to prevent the major degenerative diseases of our time. It is difficult to cure heart disease, cancer, and arthritis, but it is easy to prevent them with the proper Hildegard diet.

A good daily digestion starts with the traditional hot cereal breakfast. Coarsely ground spelt or spelt flakes are cooked in water and served with cooked apple slices spiced with cinnamon and galangal. This delicious cereal can be sweetened with honey or brown sugar and improved with ground sweet almonds. The traditional Scotch porridge—oatmeal—also meets the requirements of a warm breakfast prepared from the fruits of the field:

If a person has not yet breakfasted, the first thing he or she eats should be a food which is prepared from fruits of the field and from flour; for that is a dry food and delivers a healthy strength. In addition, he or she should eat something warm so that it heats the gastrointestinal system and, indeed, should avoid all cold foods. (CC 115, 27)

Are our age-old intuitions right about the warm breakfast, which has been customary from time immemorial, and are modern nutritional reformers wrong about a cold breakfast or appetizer? Try it and see the difference in your digestion by starting the day with a warm spelt porridge, or cold orange juice and uncooked cereal.

Spelt porridge, spelt bread, and spelt coffee constitute the ideal breakfast. Spelt coffee is a mixture of eighty percent brown-roasted and twenty percent dark-roasted spelt kernels cooked whole in water, to provide a tasty drink which stimulates a regular bowel function.

Breakfast, as the first meal of the day, stimulates a vegetative intestinal rhythm. This rhythm is supported by one's daily habits. Only rarely should they be changed. If you eat your daily breakfast at the same time, then the intestines will regularly react in the same way. Instead of coffee or cigarettes to aid digestion, it is much better to use the routine of the daily spelt coffee breakfast, which has no side effects.

Hildegard says, however, that for a healthy person it is best not to eat any breakfast at all:

For a physically healthy person it is nevertheless good and healthy to forego breakfast until before midday, or around noon, because it improves the digestion. For the sick, frail, and physically run-down, it is good and healthy to breakfast in the mornings in order at least to gain some strength from the nourishment, which one might not have had otherwise. (CC 116, 7 ff)

In order to fortify a good digestion, one should drink during meals. Most people do not drink enough; they are chronically dehydrated. This thickens all body fluids and tissues. A poor mucous lining in the gastrointestinal tract cannot lubricate and causes a slow movement of the bowels. Because of this, the normal ability of the bowels to eliminate naturally on their own is ruined completely. Drinking during meals prevents the feces from hardening and developing into constipation.

Constipation is often the result of a sick gastrointestinal tract due to bad eating habits. It is a good rule not to start any meal with fruit or salad, one of the most harmful reasons for digestive disorders like gas, foul stool, or constipation. If the stomach is offered a vegetable salad first, digestion stops and the following food remains largely indigested. Therefore, start dinner with soup, and eat salad with the rest of the meal. Herbs improve proper digestion and assist the body in throwing off accumulated toxins and waste products, furnishing good blood circulation. (PL 1126 A)

Fennel in any form, as spice, vegetable, tea, or tablets, promotes a good digestion (PL 1156 D). However eaten, fennel makes us happy, gives a healthy skin color, produces a pleasant body odor and supports a good digestion. Fennel seeds are 100-percent good for your health.

Eaten daily on an empty stomach, they reduce mucus and all rottenness, take away halitosis and clear the eyes. (PL 1156 C)

Fennel acts like an antacid, neutralizing stomach acid:

Whoever eats fried meat, fried fish, or anything else fried, and suffers pain from it should eat fennel or fennel seeds and will have less pain. (PL 1157 B)

People with poor circulation and a cold stomach (gastric stomach) cannot digest effectively and should eat field mint (*Mentha arvensis* L) either raw or cooked with meat or fish. Field mint will warm the stomach, increase blood circulation and help digestion. (PL 1161 C)

Steamed watercress (*Nasturtium officinale* L) improves poor

45

digestion. It is a great remedy for patients with jaundice and fever.

Whoever has jaundice or fever should steam watercress in a bowl, eat it often warm, and it will heal this person. And whoever can hardly digest eaten foods should likewise steam watercress in a bowl, because its energy comes from water. Eat it and it will help. (PL 1161 A)

One of the best and most effective spices, a basic in Hildegard's kitchen, is pellitory (*Anacyclus pyrethrum* L). Two or three pinches of pellitory should be cooked in each meal or added as a spice. Pellitory is responsible for an effective assimilation of nutrients by the intestines into the blood, and therefore increases the strength and health of the entire organism.

Hildegard writes about pellitory:

It is good for a healthy person to eat, because it lessens rottenness, increases the good blood, and makes a clear head. And it will even bring back strength to the sick person who came close to death, and will send nothing undigested out of the person, but rather give him or her a good digestion. (PL 1138 D)

Everyone has found that heavy food can disturb a good sleep. The secret of life is always found in the middle; anything in moderation is good for your health. The digestive tract can digest the evening meal more easily if it has already had a chance to adjust to the same food during the day. Perhaps the digestive work which follows will disturb the sleeper less with bad dreams. But do not sleep or snooze immediately after meals.

A person should not sleep right after eating, before the taste, the juice, and the smell of the foods have arrived at their destinations. Rather this person should keep himself or herself from sleeping after a meal for a short time, so that this sudden sleep does not lead the taste, juice, and smell of the foods to wrong, unsuitable body parts, and does not distribute them like dust here and there in the vessels. (CC 114, 5)

Common degenerative diseases, such as cancer, heart, and lung ailments and liver cirrhosis, are the end result of the health-destroying living and eating habits of today. The coffee and doughnuts life style is as much at fault as the cocktail-hour habit with its problems of social drinking and smoking. Hildegard presents several unfavorable factors leading to digestive disorders and intestinal diseases:

46

1. Overeating, especially overconsumption of red meat (beef).
2. Eating raw foods.
3. Improper preparation of food (canned, ultra-high-heated, sterile).
4. Eating foods too high in animal fat.
5. Eating juiceless or dry foods (refined, stripped).

About these foods which can be harmful for heart, liver, and lungs, Hildegard writes:

Therefore they curdle in the stomach, become hard and mouldy, so that they spread slime [somewhat green or blue-green or even lead-colored] in the stomach. Like a rotting manure pile, they send out bad fluids and harmful, terrible smelling fumes throughout the whole body, like when green or wet wood burns an evil smoke and circulates every-where in the body. (CC 99, 17)

Digestive disorders causing indigestion with putrefying foods, putrefactive bacteria, foul stool, flatulence, and increase of transit time in the bowels may eventually lead to dangerous intestinal diseases, including colitis, diverticulitis, and constipation. As the body becomes increasingly toxic, proper oxidation cannot take place. Without oxidation, the body is fatigued. Eating the right Hildegard diet and getting the right exercise and fresh air cleans out the intestines, develops proper bowel elimination, and restores regular bowel function.

Digestive disorders can almost always be prevented by following the spelt diet. The reaction and results of the spelt diet have been wonderful for both patient and doctor. The spelt diet is a guarantee for health, reversing in most cases the disturbed gastrointestinal tract. Spelt is an optimal food for all gastrointestinal problems, including indigestion, gas, or flatulence and nausea. Even more serious diseases like constipation, diarrhea, colitis, stomach ulcers, gastritis, hemorrhoids, as well as liver and gall bladder sicknesses, can be helped by eating spelt.

Hildegard revealed secrets of the digestive process 800 years ago in part III of her notebook, *Aphorisms*:

The food which provides growth to human tissues is digested in the first night after consumption. Food providing strength for the intestines [and endocrine glands] is assimilated on the first day after consump-

tion. . . . The food which contributes energy to the liver is digested on the second day. Foods invigorating the spleen are digested on the third day. But the food nourishing heart and blood finishes its digestion on the tenth day, because heart and blood rely on almost the same energy.

(AP III, 39)

Laxatives, with their sudden elimination, destroy the health of the intestinal tract and cause malnutrition in other organs as well.

There are many benefits coming from the Hildegard diet. Nevertheless, it is important to establish good eating habits, like eating in moderation.

Therefore a person who takes in unwholesome and unnecessary food will be nourishing bad blood. (CC 112, 36)

Vegetables and salads should always be eaten with the meals, never before or after. Thorough chewing [twenty times each bite] supplies a proper salivation for the food and is important for good digestion.

Saliva is like a good salve; like a salve that summons health.

(CC 131, 14)

Hildegard even warns against eating extremely hot foods —ones still steaming.

If the essential gastric fluid is somehow withdrawn from the digestive process, the stomach will have a poor blood circulation. Because of health-destroying body fluids, slime fills the stomach, and the food in the gastrointestinal tract solidifies. Persons suffering from this notice a weakening of their eyes, which later may lead to various illnesses:

If digestive juice is withheld because of excess juices, then the stomach will get cold, the food pulp will harden in the stomach, and in this manner the person will become sick. Those with stomach ailments as a result of insufficient digestion will suffer from a weakening of their eyes.

(AP III, 43)

What are these excess juices? Hildegard describes three health destroying body fluids: malicious humor, noxious humor, and infirm humor. Malicious humors are health-destroying body fluids which develop from forces outside of the body, like environment and nutritional mistakes (overeating, eating raw foods). Noxious humors come from the body itself and include

48

factors such as hormone disturbances and allergies causing histamine release. Infirm humors are the sick fluids originating from infections and toxic waste products.

If all these fluids overflow the body, the normal digestive process will dry out causing constipation. (AP III, 43)

Again, a change to the Hildegard spelt diet is the easiest way to heal constipation. Spelt, especially the spelt kernel, is the best kernel grain; it has high quality and is easy to digest. The following diet, high in fiber, should be used regularly:

1. **Spelt Kernel Coffee** in the morning to stimulate the bowel function.
2. **Fresh Garden Lettuce Salad** mixed with cold cooked spelt kernels.
3. **"Fleaseeds"** (*Plantago, Psyllium*): 1 tablespoon sprinkled over every meal, instead of linseeds, which are harmful and steal vitamins and calcium from the body.
4. **Spelt Roughage**: 3-5 tablets, 3 times a day, with lots of fennel tea.
5. **Whole-Grain Spelt Kernels** (flour constipates).

Spelt, as a basic and valid nutrient for healthy and sick, can even help the most fatal constipations.

Diarrhea is diarrhea no matter what the illness is named and how specific the diagnosis is. There is a whole spectrum beginning with the upset stomach characterized by vomiting and diarrhea. Travelers suffer diarrhea caused by salmonellae or mycotic action. Dysentery (diarrhea with blood and mucus) and cholera (acute disease with watery diarrhea) are both very serious sicknesses. There is diarrhea associated with poisoning and dyspepsia, when food remains undigested, as may happen among older patients. In cases of serious diarrhea, a physician should be consulted, because a radically changing bowel movement can sometimes indicate colon cancer.

One and the same mechanism is the cause for all these different diseases involving diarrhea (except cancer). Anyone suffering from this affliction will be helped within three days by the diarrhea egg, according to Hildegard, and the spelt diet. Even in the most difficult cases, where modern chemotherapy has been of no avail, the diarrhea egg will benefit.

The diarrhea egg is prepared from one baked egg yolk and a pinch of powder mixed from seventeen grams cumin and three grams white pepper; it is crumbly dry in texture. The patient should first eat a small piece of old white bread and then one tablespoon of diarrhea egg without salt. It does not taste bad and usually helps right after the first egg. Only in severe cases will there be a need for a second or third egg on the same day. (CC 200, 18)

This procedure should be repeated as many days as necessary. With dysentery, for example, the treatment will have to be continued for at least three to four days. It pays to be cautious in cases of serious infections, since a relapse is almost always worse than the first attack.

The diarrhea egg will have to be used longest of all to cure colitis, a difficult illness of the large intestine which can go on for years. Colitis patients may have up to eight to twelve bowel movements day and night and, as a result, are reduced to skin and bones. Then one must faithfully give the diarrhea egg once or twice a day for weeks or months, always preceding it with a piece of old white bread. After a while, the patient will notice with pleasure that the bowel movement becomes more and more seldom, and finally the illness is healed!

DIARRHEA DIET

First Day

The patient should only be given warm, unsweetened fennel tea to drink, as much as he or she wishes. Occasionally thin, unsweetened black tea may also be given, since it is a mild circulatory stimulant and helps solidify the stools. In acute conditions, including sickness involving fever, avoid all foods for the first three critical days.

Second Day

On the second day, some dry zwieback, matzos, or hard tack may be given. Bread made with yeast or milk is reserved for the third day.

Third Day

On the third day, a thin spelt flour cereal may be eaten. The spelt flour is simply cooked in water and slightly salted. The patient can eat as much as he or she wishes. Spelt is definitely superior to any other grain in the diet. Neither oats nor rice cereal are appropriate. As a replacement, one might try a white bread soup finely strained.

GENERAL DIARRHEA DIET
FOR FURTHER TREATMENT

The following foods are strictly forbidden during the full period of diarrhea:

1. All milk and dairy products such as cheese, cottage cheese, cream, buttermilk, ice cream. Butter is allowed in small quantities.
2. Dark bread, coarse or whole grain bread, fresh yeast bread.
3. Water and mineral water.
4. All cold food and drinks.
5. All roasted and fried food.
6. Raw food, salads, raw fruits.
7. Coarse vegetables like leeks, cucumbers, or mashed potatoes.
8. Beef, dried meat, and sausage.
9. Sugar, sugar products, jelly.
10. Hot spices like mustard, paprika, etc.

The following foods are permitted during the whole period of diarrhea:

1. White bread, whole white bread, old yeast bread, zwieback. Spelt flour and any products made from spelt: noodles, dumplings, etc.
2. Warmed wine, especially red wine.
3. Chicken and poultry.
4. Boiled apples (not apple sauce), apple cake (not too fresh).
5. Stewed veal and liver.
6. Cooked raspberries, cherries, blackberries.
7. Four to six cups of fennel tea a day.

After the condition improves, the meal can be enlarged gradually to contain the whole Hildegard diet. (See Chapter Eight for further information.)

Gastric or duodenal stomach pain, gastritis, and eventually ulceration may result from a variety of physiological and psychological factors, such as nutritional, dietary mistakes (raw food, overeating, too hot or too cold, too sour or too sweet, too much fat) or severe mental stress, frustration, and worries.

Permanent nervous and mental strain can cause a gastritis sooner or later, with or without too much gastric acid, and the possibility of stomach cancer or pernicious anemia. Therefore, the underlying psychological causes must be eliminated or removed before the Hildegard treatment can be successful. Persons with a predisposition for stomach ulcers should have an emerald stone put on the pit of the stomach, especially when atmospheric influences like weather or seasonal changes are responsible.

The Hildegard diet, with its emphasis on spelt products, is the basis of an effective treatment. Almond milk made from blanched almonds and water ground and mixed in a blender is very helpful, since it neutralizes the excess stomach acid and provides high quality proteins. Goat meat helps heal the ulcerated mucous membranes of the stomach and intestines. Goat milk also helps neutralize gastric acid.

Whoever has stomach pain should fry goat liver and eat it often until mid-August. It will heal and cleanse the stomach like a good purgative. (PL 1325 B)

The following foods must be avoided:

1. All sour fruit, especially citrus fruit.
2. Raw food.
3. All fried food, including vegetable oils.
4. Tobacco, alcohol, coffee, chocolate.
5. Strong spices, mustard, paprika.
6. Sugar and sugar products, including drinks and soft drinks.

In acute cases of active ulcers, chestnut soup in the morning is recommended for four weeks.

Whoever has a stomach ache should boil chestnuts in water and then mash them. Then this person should mix some breadcrumbs in a bowl with water and add to this mixture licorice powder and a bit less the powder of female fern [Polypodium vulgare], and cook it once more

with the chestnuts, preparing a soup. Then eat of it and it will clean the
stomach, making it warm and strong. (PL 1227 B)

Halitosis can come either from the mouth, the nose and
throat cavity, the bronchial system, i.e. the lungs, or it can be
emitted from the circulatory system into the exhaled air. Digestion produces fifteen quarts of gas every day! In all of these cases
fennel in the form of tablets or seeds has proved to be a good
remedy. Fennel seeds contain two to six percent essential oil,
which is responsible for its cleansing and mildly disinfecting
properties. For heartburn and belching, fennel is also a reliable
and safe remedy, so that I call it the "Tagamed" of Hildegard
medicine.

NAUSEA & VOMITING
AS A SIMPLE ILLNESS
& in cases of pregnancy & travel sickness

Hildegard describes an easy and effective treatment for the
person who suffers from a predisposition for nausea with vomiting, called the cumin/egg yolk cookies (*Pulvis cuminum cyninum
compositum*) and cumin bread treatment.

*Those who suffer from nausea should take cumin [thirty grams] and
a third part of white pepper [ten grams] as well as the fourth part of
cumin pimpernel [8½ grams,* Pimpinella saxifraga] *as a powder,
together with flour and egg yolk; add some water, form cookies, and bake
them. Eat the cookies as well as the cumin powder on a piece of bread.*
(PL 1138 A)

The cumin/egg yolk cookies are prepared as follows: Add
one to two teaspoons of cumin compositum powder to 100 grams
flour and a bit of salt and sugar. Mix this with six to eight egg
yolks and with as little water as possible to make a dough, which
can be formed and baked. The egg yolk cookies must be baked
at a medium temperature (350-400°F).

The treatment for nausea and vomiting is as follows:

1. Eat several of the egg yolk cookies a day.

2. Eat a piece of bread sprinkled with cumin compositum powder, chew well.

As the condition improves, the amount of egg yolk cookies
can be gradually reduced. Through this treatment, the trigger

53

center in the brain which controls nausea is properly adjusted and the problem is solved for cases of simple vomiting.

Habitual vomiting is most common among children and young people. In the case of school children, one should not look upon it as simply a bad habit, an error in upbringing, or a "complex." The children are usually happy to be freed from their "nightmares" with the cumin treatment. Afterwards they will be better able to master conflicts just like other children. To avoid being seasick or travel sick, the treatment must be given somewhat ahead of time. This simple persistent tendency to nausea, which usually begins in childhood, makes up more than half of the complaints of this sort.

One can use this method in cases of simple morning sickness associated with pregnancy, without worrying about harming the unborn child. Pregnancy is not a real illness, but its nausea can be alleviated with the use of cumin/egg yolk cookies, which, by the way, also satisfy the craving for spicy things. On the other hand, sausages and the like should be immediately and completely avoided in any problem pregnancies. The consumption of meat should be limited as much as possible. The need for protein should be met through other foods (cheese, milk, cottage cheese, almonds).

Vomiting is often a result of chemical irritations caused by the toxic effects of bacterial or mycotic action, toxins during pregnancy, decomposition material caused by X-ray treatment, or as a defense of the male sperm. Irritations may also be traced to overeating, eating the wrong food combinations, overindulgence in rich foods or alcohol, eating too fast, or eating too much fat. The most common psychological reason for vomiting is the unresolved problem of dislike or rejection of things or persons that one does not want to see or accept. (She's sick of him!)

Before the treatment of vomiting which results from a serious illness or accident, a physician should be consulted. Such underlying illnesses stand in the foreground and include migraine, high fever infections, poisoning, gall bladder inflammation, appendicitis, and severe pain in or around one eye in cases of acute glaucoma and jaundice. Recurrent vomiting caused by persistent inflammation of the stomach lining, or ulceration; suffering from recurrent headaches with pressure on the brain, or as a result of bleeding or a tumor; and vomiting with red or black blood, as a result of damage to the lining of the esophagus, also require immediate medical treatment.

Most other cases of vomiting can be effectively treated at home with cumin/egg yolk cookies. Providing that no serious illnesses are suspected, these additional self-help measures are worth a try:

1. Eat no solid food except the eggyolk cookie until vomiting and nausea have subsided and do not forget bread sprinkled with cumin powder as part of the treatment.

2. Drink plenty of fennel or thin black tea in small sips, even if you cannot keep anything else down.

3. Do not smoke or drink alcohol; take no aspirin!

4. If nauseated, lie down until the sensation fades.

Most patients with gastritis, which mainly causes stomach pains in elderly persons, have a deficiency of gastric digestive juices. They and others with temporarily poor digestion can be helped by taking one tablespoon of clary sage (*Salvia sclarea*) stomach tonic after each meal. Good digestion is very important to good health. (PL 1191 B)

In Hildegard's book, *Book of Life's Merits*, the grotesque figure of the Glutton speaks:

God created everything. Why should I lack anything? Had God not known that man needs all this, God would not have made it. I would be crazy if I couldn't follow my pleasure and enjoy all these wonderful things, particularly because God wants each person to take the responsibility for his or her bodily well-being. (LVM II)

To which Abstinence answers:

No one plays the zither so that its strings break! If all the strings break at once, what would remain of the sound? Nothing at all! You stuff your belly so full, you glutton, that your veins almost burst and writhe in cramps. Where is there a trace of the sweet sound of truth, which God bestowed on humankind? Deaf and blind you are and you don't know what to say. (LVM II)

I create a standard in humankind, so that the body lacks nothing, but also doesn't become too voluptuous, stuffed full of food and drink, much more than needed. I am a zither that sounds with the most beautiful music and in its goodwill penetrates hard hearts. Whenever an individual cares for the body reasonably, then I play intercessions on the zither for him or her in heaven. And as long as the body is refreshed through nourishment in moderation, I sing to the harp.

But you, Glutton, you know nothing of these things and don't even once try to see and understand them. One time you plunge into improper fasting, so that you can barely stay alive. Another time you stuff your belly so full in your greed that you boil over and must vomit vile slime.

But I take only enough nourishment that the juices of the organism do not dry out and thereby get out of balance, and in this way I praise to the zither and sing to the organ.   (LVM II)

Chapter Eight

DIET

YOU ARE
WHAT YOU EAT

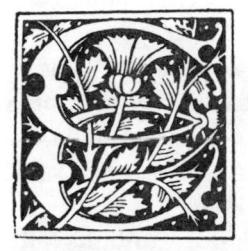verything you eat and drink either strengthens or harms your health and vitality, just as your positive or negative thoughts strengthen or harm your spirit. But how do we know what strengthens or weakens us? Hildegard shows us a nutritional way to better health as presented in detail in the book, *The Kitchen Secrets of Hildegard's Medicine*. Hildegard's diet is superior to the many contradictory man-made diets of today, because of its divine origin.

Proper nutrition is more important than medicine, including drugs, surgery and physiotherapy. The spelt diet, especially, builds and maintains healthy cells, good blood, tissues, glands, organs and body functions, and even a happy mind and a joyful spirit. Orthodox medicine is not the best hope for future health; it is diet that will define our destiny. This is reflected in the inconsistent recommendation of a famous university hospital to a sixteen-year-old patient suffering from colitis, that he take fifty milligrams of cortisone daily and eat whatever he wanted. Finally, to the surprise of his doctors, he did recuperate after following Hildegard's diet and reducing his cortisone intake.

The "eat anything you want" theory has brought us a tremendous number of degenerative diseases. Today it is generally recognized that many of the first ten killers of modern society are linked to diet, among these:

heart disease   diabetes

57

cancer   cirrhosis of the liver
stroke   circulatory disease
lung disease   emotional & physical stress
influenza

It is much easier to prevent these diseases through the Hildegard diet than to treat them.

The Hildegard diet is based on *viriditas*, or the life energy found in nature. This life energy is able to rejuvenate our cells and keep us alive. The secret of life itself is found in the cereal grain, spelt, the heart of the whole Hildegard diet.

Hildegard admires spelt over every other grain, writing:

Spelt is the best grain; it is warming, fattening, strengthening, has a high quality, and is milder than any other grain. Spelt produces firm flesh and good blood, provides a happy mind and a joyful spirit. No matter how you eat spelt, either as a bread or in other foods, it is good and easy to digest. (PL 1131 C)

You might not find this little grain on your market shelf yet, but spelt is the food of the future.

Spelt has been thoroughly analyzed and contains all required nutrients: proteins of high biological value (essential amino acids), fatty acids (lipids) for the nervous system, carbohydrates, vitamins, a gold mine of minerals, and a rich source of dietary fiber.

Spelt, as the basic food, provides a constant energy flow, because the carbohydrate chain is slowly broken down in the intestine, molecule by molecule, and is burned completely, leaving water and carbon dioxide, which are easily eliminated. You will not feel as tired or as emotionally drained as you do when you eat denatured, refined grain—the so-called "empty calories," i.e. white sugar in candy, and white flour in bread. Refined starch and sugar are immediately assimilated into the blood—not broken down like spelt—causing a "high" or rush of energy which is quickly burned, leaving no sugar in the blood. This is what causes hypoglycemia, or low blood sugar, hyperactive children, or even obesity. The "empty calories" are being stored as body fat, while the body is starving to death for a lack of all essential nutrients.

The simplicity of the Hildegard diet does not require measuring the complicated data of calorie charts, vitamin tables, fat percentages, or fiber content. This simple diet is totally complete. Supplementation through additional vitamin or mineral pills is not only unnecessary, but is not recommended. Hildegard's frugal diet contains fresh vegetables and fruits in season, preferably grown in the immediate area. Instead of an overabundance of various foods from exotic lands, and the cultivation of gourmet tastes, Hildegard advocates a plain diet which can nevertheless be delicious and healthful.

The characteristic, important, and fundamental substance of a food is its essence (essential), its subtility. For the Hildegard diet, this is the scale which weighs and selects the foods. On the basis of subtility we can select "good" foods from the various food families for our diet. All things 100-percent "good" have health-promoting, health-sustaining, rejuvenating, and vitalizing qualities as a part of their fundamental nature.

WHOLE GRAINS

1. Spelt:
the most ancient grain—the very best; use for cooking and baking.
2. Oats:
only good for healthy persons; promotes beautiful skin; leads to health and happiness. (PL 1130 C)
3. Wheat:
only good as wholewheat or graham, and only for baking.
4. Rye:
only good for healthy persons; excellent for those who tend to have heavy fat deposits (hard workers); detrimental for persons with weak stomachs (gastritis). (PL 1130 A)
5. Barley:
injures healthy persons and those with anemia and poor circulation, for barley lacks the values which are found in the other grains. (PL 1131 B)

RECOMMENDED VEGETABLES

1. Beans:

green beans, soy beans, kidney beans, all other beans.

2. Fennel:
however eaten, fennel makes us happy, produces beautiful skin, good digestion, and good body odor.

3. Celery:
cooked.

4. Chickpeas

5. Pumpkin

6. Watercress

7. Red Beets

8. Lettuce:
only with dressing; strengthens the brain and provides good digestion.

9. Chestnuts:
fill empty brain; strengthen heart, liver, and stomach.

10. Onions:
cooked.

11. Corn-on-the-Cob

12. Broccoli

RECOMMENDED FRUITS

1. Apples:
raw for healthy only; cooked or well baked for sick and healthy; old, wrinkled, raw apples also good for sick.

2. Cherries

3. Quince:
especially good for rheumatism and arthritis.

4. Red and Black Currants

5. Grapes

6. Raspberries, Blackberries

7. Citrus Fruits

8. Cornel Cherries

9. Melons

10. Dates:
in moderation.

MEATS

1. Fish:
good for healthy and sick—pike, perch, roach, and grayling.
good only for healthy—salmon, herring, carp, and trout.

2. Poultry & Chicken:
easy to digest; Hildegard recommends its use all year round; prepare without skin.
turkey—though Hildegard is silent on turkey, it is easy to digest and is lowest in cholesterol of all meats.
wild goose, wild duck—only for the healthy.
ostrich meat—excellent for obese persons.

3. Lamb:
in spring and summer; good for healthy and sick; especially good for varicose veins. Hildegard writes:

Whoever is failing in his whole body and whose veins are withered should often sip the juice of lamb and of the soup in which it was cooked. Also he should eat some of the meat and, when he improves, he can eat even more meat if he wants. (PL 1324 A)

4. Goat:
in spring and summer; good for healthy and sick. In Hildegard's words:

If goat meat is eaten often, it heals obstructed and malfunctioning weakened intestines and heals and strengthens the stomach. (PL 1325 A)

5. Venison:
in fall and winter; good for healthy and sick. Hildegard says:

Whoever eats of this meat frequently is cleansed of slime and filth. Whoever is plagued by precancerosis [vicht] should eat often from its liver and it will devour the vicht in him. (PL 1321 D)

DRESSINGS AND SPICES

The standard dressing for Hildegard's salad contains one tablespoon pure wine vinegar, three tablespoons sunflower oil, and a bit of little brown sugar to neutralize the sour taste. Lemon juice, as well as yoghurt, can also be used.

ABC of Hildegard's spices:
basil
bay leaves
caraway
chervil
cinnamon—*universal spice for sinuses*
cloves
cubeb pepper—*clears the intellect*

cumin—*makes cheese more digestible*
curled mint
dill
fennel—*"happy-making" spice, good for bad breath*
galangal—*activates entire organism, especially heart*
garlic
horseradish
hyssop—*chicken spice; excellent for liver colic and melancholy*
lovage
marjoram
mother of thyme—*good for skin disorders*
mugwort
nutmeg
oregano
parsley
pellitory—*universal spice; aids digestion of all nutrients*
pimpernel
rosemary
rue
sage
savory
stinging nettle
watercress
watermint

BEVERAGES

Hildegard recommends that one drink in moderation during the meal.

The best tea is fennel tea, which is 100-percent good for your health. You can also use lemon balm or rosehips for your tea.

Beer is a beverage especially good for the underweight. It is a good muscle builder and provides a healthy skin color.

Wine is also good in moderation—almost a remedy for the sick. But do not forget to add a squirt of water in order to "humanize" the wine. The quenched wine is especially helpful to keep you happy. (See Chapter Eleven.)

Spelt coffee, a roasted-grain coffee substitute, is recommended for the digestion, especially as a breakfast coffee.

Spring and well water are normally better than mineral water. As a general rule, a good mineral water should contain as few minerals as possible, in order to cleanse the body of waste products. Mineral water is not always good as a main drink, especially if it contains too many minerals.

Orange and lemon juice are good for your health, especially when fever is present.

DIET FOR THE SICK

First Stage

On the first day, in the acute stage of a disease, when fever is present, total fasting is recommended. Do not eat; only drink the best tea. Fennel tea is especially beneficial to one's health, as is rose-hip tea. In cases of high fever without diarrhea, particularly with viral infection in summer or fall, a glass of water with galangal (*Alpinia galanga*) will take care of the fever. When diarrhea is involved, one can drink a weak black tea. Occasionally, one can eat some zwieback dipped into tea. This is also beneficial on the second day with chunks of cooked apples, but not mashed apples. Cooked apples are more easily digested than raw apples for sick people—as are pears, which we do not suggest for sick people.

On the second day, one may have a cream-of-spelt soup, spiced with a little salt and parsley. A spelt-flour soup is suggested for diarrhea sufferers, but do not eat soup from oats, barley, or rice, which causes constipation and is difficult to digest. Spelt dumplings and noodles are also good.

If there is no diarrhea on the third day, one can eat chicken bouillon and chicken without skin. Quenched wine is also a good idea. Fruits other than apples are not necessary, because the apple meets all your needs in the first three days. This diet is suggested also for recurrent back problems.

Second Stage

On the fourth day of an illness, a diet of the following foods is recommended: wholewheat bread, old yeast bread, and spelt bread of all kinds; fruits recommended above, all stewed; meat and vegetables recommended above. To the spelt dishes recommended for the second day, one may add oat porridge (with chopped almonds), noodles, spelt flakes (porridge), and cream-of-spelt soup.

63

In addition, a poached egg without the egg white, well-chopped salad with dressing (see above), biscuits, zwieback, apple cake (not too sweet), and spelt coffee or fennel tea to drink are recommended. No chocolate, no ice cream!

Third Stage

A diet for long-term disease is recommended for the chronically ill and persons suffering from arthritis or rheumatism. All is permitted, except the following:

Bologna, mayonnaise, fried eggs in the evening; cheese, but with cumin spice; canned food, sardines, eel, shrimp, kelp, pork, margarine, duck or goose.

Strawberries, peaches, plums, and leeks (the famous four-season poisons); cucumbers, blueberries, pears (especially if suffering with migraine, diarrhea, or colds).

Rhubarb, walnuts, or potatoes; alcoholic beverages (except beer and wine), coffee or tobacco; whipped cream or pommes frites (french fries).

Do not eat foods that are too hot, too cold, too sweet, or too bitter.

Chapter Nine

LIVER

BLACK BILE &
DEPRESSION

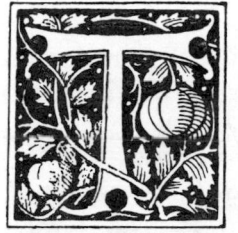

he liver is like a bowl in a person into which heart, lungs, and stomach pour their juices, which the liver in turn lets flow back to all members of the body, just as any container placed under a fountain will let the water received flow out elsewhere. But if the liver is full of holes and fragile, it will be unable to absorb the good juices from heart, lungs, and stomach. These juices and liquids return back to the heart, lungs, and stomach and cause there a kind of flood. If this sickness ever begins in a person, he or she will not be able to live long.

(CC 98, 10)

With this comparison, Hildegard describes the circulation of the portal vein, which causes blood from the liver to flow back to the heart and, from there, on into the lungs. Where did Hildegard get her knowledge about the liver and its function? The doctors of her time knew nothing about liver metabolism and nothing at all about the circulation of the portal vein. Nor did the abbess find out through her own research that the liver is supplied and purified through the liver artery with arterial blood, as well as through the portal vein with venous blood.

The liver is, as we know today, a wonderful workshop. In it, building materials plus energy for muscles and work are stored, made ready, and converted into action. Its main function is supplying the blood with nutrients, such as proteins, carbohydrates, and fat, and utilizing them. The liver stores sugar (glucose), or changes excess sugar quantities into fat. If required, the liver can change it back into sugar, as between mealtimes, during sports, or as an important supplier of energy for the brain.

Protein is divided into its original building blocks by the liver, out of which the body builds its own body protein. Hereby the body's own substance is formed from these original building blocks according to the holy construction plan inherent in every person, which scientists call the genetic code.

Like a filter, the liver removes harmful waste products and pollutants like alcohol, nicotine, or chemical medicines from the blood. These are changed into water-soluble, unpoisonous substances, so that the kidneys can excrete them. Through too many poisons and wastes, the liver can become so swamped that the "filter" obstructs and the liver either swells or is destroyed.

In addition, the dead blood corpuscles, which were decomposed by the spleen, are changed by the liver into bile (bilirubin) and eliminated with gallic acid produced by the liver. This yellow bile is supplied to the duodenum for the digestion of fats, producing the brown-colored urobilinogen in the intestine, which gives stool its color. Disturbances in the bile production will color stool pale or light grey, whereby urine becomes dark brown, since the bile has to be eliminated with the urine. The bilirubin level rising in the blood colors the skin yellow (quince) by jaundice. Excess bile is stored in the gall bladder, concentrated, and on demand, as by heavy meals, delivered to the intestine. Now black bile is formed. In Hildegard medicine, black bile has a great importance and causes not only severe inner sicknesses, but also negative moods.

Based on her vision, Hildegard's knowledge does not relate only to the science of biochemistry. More than any other person, she saw the key to health or sickness in the passions of mankind. Sadness and anger are the results of a metabolic sickness, whereby especially the metabolism of the liver can be influenced through the sense of hearing. Hearing and liver are in direct relationship with one another. (See Chapter Two.)

Ancient doctors were familiar with healing by means of music. Today, music therapy can open a heart or normalize liver metabolism in depressed patients through singing, dancing, or simply through listening.

Hildegard also knew that liver diseases and depressions can be traced back to inherited characteristics, or can be dependant on the moment of conception:

There are also persons who were conceived by the waning moon and under the turbulence of changing air currents. Some of them are always sad and have a restless character. Because of their sadness, their liver becomes weakened and perforated by many very tiny holes like cheese. Therefore, such persons do not eat much and have no desire for food and drink, but rather eat and drink with restraint. Because they eat and drink so little, their liver becomes fragile like a sponge and shrinks.

(CC 97, 37 ff)

Hildegard's description corresponds to our impression and observation of depressed patients, for whom the joy of life and its activities have so vanished that they sit there discouraged, with no appetite and motionless. Their whole metabolism is reduced to zero. The liver cells shrink and disintegrate. This is the picture of a liver atrophy. Through the shrinkage of the liver, circulation is also impeded, and this can cause a congestion in the portal vein area.

Other persons who were conceived by the full moon are so healthy that they can eat everything all mixed up. But even they can suffer from a liver disease.

Those persons who were conceived by full moon and moderately warm weather, neither too warm nor too cold, are healthy and greedy at mealtimes, eating various foods indiscriminately and in utter confusion. Although they can consume diverse foods with no choice, they should, however, hold back from some harmful [noxii] foods, like a hunter who lets unprofitable wildlife go and catches only profitable game.

(CC 97, 17 ff)

Hildegard knows the true causes of liver sicknesses. Especially through overeating, liver metabolism and the complete basic metabolism of the body can break down, as one observes with rheumatism or cancer.

If one of these [conceived by full moon] takes in different meals immoderately and without careful selection, then the liver will be harmed and hardened through the various kinds of juices in these foods. Then its healing juice, which it should have sent into all organs, single joints, and intestines, like a salve, will spoil through different harm-

67

ful juices, whereby it sometimes occurs that the flesh of this person grows into a tumor somewhere on the limbs and the tissue becomes brittle. Thereby some limb may become so damaged that the person limps on it [arthrosis deformans]. (CC 97, 25 ff)

This is the reason why basal metabolism, with special consideration for the liver, must be treated for all severe civilization sicknesses, in order to cure the fundamental disease. Besides the cleansing and detoxification measures of Hildegard medicine (bloodletting, cupping, sauna, change of diet to spelt), a person should recognize his or her limits and avoid those things that cause fatty liver or liver cirrhosis.

Hildegard often describes metabolic disturbances as the cause of liver sicknesses, whereby bad juices (*mali humores*), harmful juices (*noxi humores*) and disease-related infection juices (*infirmi humores*) confuse the complete metabolism. Sometimes a person suffers for years from bad juices, without being able to find the real cause.

Sometimes the aforementioned juices can pour into the chest of the person in profusion and eventually overflow the liver too. Excessive and diverse brooding arises in such a person, so that the person thinks he or she is going crazy. Thereupon these juices ascend to the brain, invade it, and then go back again to the stomach and cause fever. In this way a person can also become sick over a long period of time. (LDO 64)

In no medical book in the world can allergic persons find themselves so well described as in Hildegard's works, where the relationship between metabolism and the psychological causes of illness can be found.

Through these particular floodings, the intestines begin to move around the navel of the individual. Juices ascend in this manner to the brain and make the person angry. If they also upset the vessels of the loins area, then they will affect the black bile, so that the person becomes confused and falls into an unmotivated sadness. (LDO 64-65)

Persons who have various complaints like asthma, chronic fatigue, eczema with fever and headaches, without being able to find a cause, do not have to be hypochondriacs any more. Perhaps they are simply suffering from a faulty metabolism through environmental stress and poor nutrition.

THE TREATMENT OF LIVER PAIN
& CHRONIC SUFFERING OF THE LIVER

It is especially impressive to see that chronic liver damage can be successfully cured through fasting. The liver transaminases begin to normalize after one to two weeks of fasting, and a surprising regeneration of the liver takes place. A liver patient should begin treatment with fasting and the simple spelt diet. Hildegard's special liver diet emphasizes, besides spelt, such foods as chestnuts, wine vinegar, ham with wine, the spice hyssop, and almonds.

Liver pain and chronic suffering of the liver are often a result of a severe liver infection, or a poisoned liver through alcohol, tobacco, or medicines, or even through immoderate eating. The loss of one's own moderation as seen in too much eating, or the over-consumption of drugs or alcohol, damages the liver. Damaged fatty liver can eventually lead to liver cirrhosis. Due to various internal diseases, such as cancer, rheumatism, sugar diabetes, or lung afflictions, the liver also swells and is sensitive to pressure. Whoever wants to be healthy again must recognize his or her own limits and learn to live within them.

Most liver infections are caused by viral infections. Hildegard explains that the lungs are harmed continuously by disturbances in the liver metabolism. This corresponds with today's anatomical knowledge that the blood from the liver flows first to the lungs to be processed. The slightest disorder in liver metabolism means that falsely composed liver blood reaches the lungs and causes pathological phenomena there. A few liver remedies from Hildegard medicine are able to heal the lungs simultaneously. The best example is the treatment of the chronic cough on the basis of an old liver affliction using hart's tongue fern elixir.

The hart's tongue fern [scolopendrium vulgare] is warm and helps the liver, the lungs, and the painful inner organs. Take and boil it in wine, add pure honey and boil it again. Add long pepper and twice as much cinnamon powder to the prepared wine and boil once again. Strain it through a cloth to obtain a clear drink. Drink often after eating, as well as before eating, and it will benefit the liver, heal the painful inner organs, cleanse the lungs, and take away inner decay and slime.

69

(PL 1142 A/B)

The production of hart's tongue fern elixir is difficult because hart's tongue fern is protected by nature conservation.

To begin with, the patient takes one tiny glass after eating every day. Later, after one has become used to the characteristic taste, the dosage is increased to one tiny glass before and after eating for four to six weeks. The elixir cleanses the poisoned liver and lungs, eliminating the inner decay and slime, and is the most important medicine for long-standing liver afflictions, chronic bronchitis, as well as disturbances of hormone regulation. Even chronic sicknesses, like bladder infections, gall bladder infections, ovary infections, and a constant discharge, can be successfully treated with hart's tongue fern elixir. Also with asthma, one of the most difficult sicknesses to treat according to Hildegard, a try with hart's tongue fern elixir is worthwhile.

All internal diseases with pressure, or a congested feeling and pain on the right-hand side of the ribs, should be treated with fasting followed by a strict spelt diet. Correctly performed bloodletting (using the liver vein) is a part of effective treament.

More than any other organ, the liver suffers from excesses— the opposite of discretion—especially extravagance in eating, drinking, and a foolish way of life. Therefore the following dietary instructions are important to observe: not too hot and not too cold, not too sweet and not too sour; no greasy foods like French fries, lard, or whipping cream; no coffee, alcohol, or nicotine. Every food a person enjoys should be tempered with a little wine vinegar before eating, because the warmth and strength of the vinegar constrict the liver.

The person should also chew wholewheat bread well and make a sandwich out of sliced, dry ham and pour a little wine over it. The dry juice of the ham will be driven out by the warmth of the wine and bread, and in this way the tempered bread will cause the liver to constrict, so that it does not swell. (CC 176, 33 ff)

A ham sandwich helps liver patients who are tired and dizzy in the morning, as can be observed in extreme cases after hepatitis. For the health of the liver, high-grade protein is necessary like that found in spelt, the ideal food, or in sweet almonds. Because brewer's yeast contains proteins for liver patients and in

70

addition is rich in vitamin B, the recent production of spelt-bran-yeast tablets is a valuable contribution. Of these one takes three to five tablets with plenty of liquid three times a day.

Great powers of healing are found in the chestnut, not only for liver afflictions, but also for weak conditions of any kind.

The chestnut tree is very warm and because of this warmth possesses great power, since it symbolizes discretion. Everything in it and its fruit is useful against any weakness in humankind...

If the liver hurts, crush chestnut kernels and lay them in honey. These should be eaten often with this honey and the liver will get better.

(PL 1227 B)

Based on its contents and stored sun energy, the chestnut is able to completely nourish a person in a well-balanced way, so that the radiance and power of resistance are restored. Thereby it helps the liver to become healthy again and brings the person into the right harmony. The chestnut is to trees what fennel is to plants: 100-percent healthy from root to crown. In the fruit, shells, leaves, and bark are valuable substances (tamine and bioflavonoids). The fruits contain starch (45-58 percent) and protein (four to seven percent) which are special suppliers of energy for liver and nerve cells. Besides that, the fruits contain specific active substances (gaba, biogene aminic acids, neurotransmitters) necessary for nerve connections and muscle agitation, plus vitamins A, B, and C. Chestnuts can be recommended for diabetics because they contain no glucose or fructose (100 grams equals 210 calories equals 880 joules).

With ready-made chestnut flour, which is very difficult to make oneself, thirty percent chestnut honey is prepared, providing liver patients with a remedy which heals chronic liver afflictions. A patient should take one teaspoon of chestnut honey in the morning and another teaspoon in the afternoon for at least two months. Later, one should continue to eat a teaspoon of chestnut honey often. This treatment leads to healing of the liver, whereby the transaminases (the liver enzymes which enter the blood during a liver infection) are normalized again.

Another liver remedy from Hildegard is lavender-flower wine, which overcomes not only liver pain but also the feeling of pressure in a congested liver. In addition, it often relieves the lungs which are congested simultaneously, and refreshes and frees the spirit. Hildegard suggests boiling wild lavender flowers (*Lavendula officinalis*) in wine. This unsweetened lavender wine is drunk in little sips during the day for a period of six to eight weeks. If wine is not wanted, the lavender flowers may be boiled in water and honey and taken the same way. Lavender wine contains at the most two percent alcohol, because through its preparation the alcohol is boiled away. It is bitter, but so is a liver complaint.

Hildegard describes lavender as good:

...and its warmth is healthy. Whoever cooks lavender with wine, or if the person has no wine, with honey and water, and drinks it often lukewarm, it will alleviate the pain in the liver and in the lungs and the steam in his chest. Lavender wine will provide the person with pure knowledge and a clear understanding. (PL 1140 C)

Liver patients are often very sad, but they can use hyssop, a happy-making spice. Hyssop is an ideal spice cooked with chicken, or in wine as a drink.

If one eats hyssop often, one cleans the sick-makers and stinkiness out of the foamy juices. . . Hyssop is good in all foods. It is more useful powdered and cooked than raw. It makes the liver active and cleanses the lungs somewhat. But if the liver is sick because of the person's sadness, the person should cook young chicken with hyssop before the sickness increases. The person should often eat this hyssop and chicken, and should also eat fresh hyssop laid in wine, and then drink the wine.

(PL 1156 AC)

In conclusion, it is good for liver patients to eat five to ten sweet almonds every day. Almonds are a kind of universal remedy to strengthen the nerves, provide a good complexion, drive away headaches, invigorate the lungs, and heal the liver.

Whoever has an empty brain and a bad complexion, and therefore headache, should eat almonds often and they will fill up the brain and give the right coloring. Also, whoever is lung sick and has liver damage should eat almonds raw or cooked often and they will bring strength to the lungs, because they do not burden or dry out a person in any way, but provide strength. (PL 1225 CD)

The various liver diseases have causes described by Hildegard, which are closely related to both the metabolism of the liver and to that of the whole body. A person who strains his or her energy through a foolish way of life will have liver problems. The liver likewise suffers, if the capacity for work is overestimated. Sadness or depression and the resulting escape into overactivity, as well as loud-mouthed inappropriate laughter, can harm the liver. Improper and ill-timed pleasure is out of place for the individual and for the liver.

Every person who overestimates his or her limits, abilities, and strength through too much food, too much alcohol, too many drugs, etc., falls from the middle way. Hildegard lists results of this imbalance as roaming thoughts, tiredness, weakness, fluttering of the heart, senseless sadness, and an inner lack of resistance, none of which leads to anything good. In her last theological book, *Liber Divinorum Operum*, Hildegard writes that every person has the name and the appointed measure assigned by God, and that the soul demands moderation in all things "because humanity cannot constantly live in heavenly heights. But the devil does not want such keeping within bounds; the devil aims for excesses, whether it be the highest or the lowest."

By avoiding greasy foods and being obedient, one can follow the way of healing and obtain discretion. Out of a bright cloud, Discretia shines towards the fiery power of God. With a bouquet of flowers, she scares away the suggestions of the devil like mosquitoes. The power of God strengthens her on her right shoulder as a cross, and in her lap she carefully and lovingly watches over the virtues like precious stones. She says:

All things that stand in God's order correspond with one another. The stars sparkle from the light of the moon, and the moon shines from the fire of the sun. Everything serves a higher purpose, and nothing exceeds its measure. (LVM II, 21)

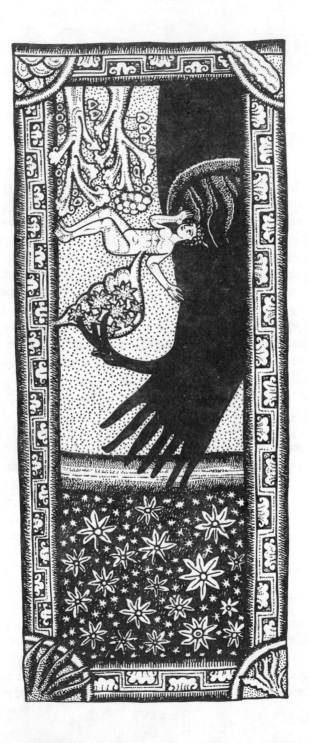

Chapter Ten

GALL BLADDER
JAUNDICE
& MELANCHOLY

ince paradise in the Garden of Eden, humans have lost their ability to enjoy, untroubled, the beautiful and the good. At the moment of their fall into sin, evil stole into their body and caused the original, shining, crystal-clear gallstone of the knowledge of God to become liquid. Since this time their gall bladder overflows and poisons their blood, so that they fall into sickness-making passions such as sadness, anger, rage, frustration, resentment, and worries. Because Adam knew good, but did evil, he fell into sickness-making conflicts. In similar situations, humans remember their origins and find protection from evil in the fear of God. Out of the knowledge of good and evil, and the understanding that you are a human and responsible to God, comes the great strength to avoid evil and do good! (SC, 10th vision)

In the same moment when Adam violated God's commandment, the bile collected in his blood; similarly the brightness goes away as soon as the light is turned off. When the brilliance was extinguished in him, black bile coagulated in his blood, out of which sadness and doubt developed. The devil hoarded up so much black bile in Adam that it made humankind into doubters and unbelievers. Because humans are such that they cannot exceed their own limits, they fear God, are sad, and finally sink into despair, no longer believing that God protects them.

Since humans are created in God's likeness, they have no

choice but to fear God. Since humans fear God more than the
devil, they put their hope in God, so that the devil cannot seize
them. But often the suggestions of the devil force their way into
humans through the black bile and make them sad and desper-
ate, so that many of them suffocate in their desperation and condemn themselves. Many others, however, resist this evil so
fiercely that they are victorious like martyrs. (CC 143, 22 ff)

Hildegard explains how humankind wants to glorify itself
through its vanity and, instead of fearing God, strives for tran-
sient prestige and admiration, saying: "Only with Lucifer can we
achieve great glory!" Hildegard pictures this love of fame (*inanis
gloria*) as a figure comparable to a modern-day conductor dressed
in tailcoat, the symbol of craving for the world's applause.
Humankind can free itself from this passion through fasting, in
order to acquire the healing fear of God.

In the passions of humankind, Hildegard sees the key to
either health or sickness. The happy or sad-making principle is
determined through the chemical balance of bile and black bile
(melanche). The bitter bite of black bile can drive humans into
the darkness of ungodliness. Sadness and anger befall and torture a person with pain like piercing nails, until his or her excess
bile disappears again.

If humans did not possess the bitterness of bile and the darkness of
black bile, they would always be healthy.   (CC 146, 27)

With scientific exactness, Hildegard describes the biochemical processes involved in an outburst of anger, a gout attack, or
a rheumatic attack. In addition, she explains methods with
which one can find one's way out of these disturbances. Melancholy must be removed in a person, if anger is not to develop.
Hildegard presents a long list of happy-making remedies, which
can neutralize the excess black bile and overcome evil. (See
antimelancholica in Chapter Eleven.)

Since the devil hates the power of virtues in humans, he also hates
all creation which possesses strong healing powers. Whether hidden in
animals or in plants, this healing power is useful and beautiful.
                                                              (CC 144, 18 ff)

Everything healthy, everything restorative, living, and beautiful has the happy-making quality, whether it is the fragrance

76

of a rose, a beautiful meal, or a precious stone. Some happy-makers useful for gall bladder patients are aloe water, diamond water, quenched wine, and the chalcedony stone.

In every person whose bile is stronger than black bile, his or her anger is more easily subdued. But if the black bile is stronger than the bile, the person will tend to anger and will become mad more easily. Just as strong sour vinegar comes from good wine, so the bile will increase from good, tasty foods and decrease through bad juices. The black bile, on the other hand, decreases from good tasty foods. From bad, bitter-tasting, unclean and poorly prepared foods, as well as from various sickness-making juices during severe sicknesses, the concentration of black bile will increase. (CC 146, 29 ff)

Anger is personified by Hildegard as a naked being stuck in the spokes of a mill wheel. The whites of the eyes swell out over the pupils as this being desperately tries to move the wheel with grasshopper arms and legs. In fury, this being has no self-respect nor respect for others, but follows only inner drives. Even the angry, wise person rages in senseless fury, and the angry, patient person degenerates into impatience and a lack of moderation. Because the person loses all understanding during an outburst of anger, he or she destroys every good seed within. As soon as anger takes power over a person, this person gets off track and is led into such a senseless raging that he or she thinks neither on heavenly nor on earthly things.

If black bile is not neutralized, the anger in a person will speak:

I crush and destroy everything that is in my way. With the sword I strike around me, and with the club I blast it all! (LVM I, 22)

Only with fasting can the angry person come back to patience, and only with Patience can the blossoms and fruits of the virtues grow, because she provides time for growth and says:

Whatever I begin, I will see it through. I will persevere faithfully and destroy no one... (LVM I, 23)

Through an excess of bile, jaundice is sometimes created, especially when the bile ducts are obstructed. This is not the so-called infectious hepatitis, for which treatment belongs in the hands of a doctor or hospital. This is the noninfectious jaundice which may be caused by a disorder of the gall bladder or liver. It begins with the typical yellow discoloration of the skin and eyes as the most prominent symptoms.

The affliction known as jaundice results from an overabundance of bile. Excess bile is produced by diseased humors, fever, and by frequent bouts of extreme rage. This effusion of bile is absorbed by the liver and the other viscera. It also penetrates and injures the flesh of the entire body, just as a strong vinegar penetrates a new keg. Thus it is that jaundice can be recognized by its unusual color. (CC 155, 3)

Those who have jaundice should put aloe (Aloe vulgaris) *in cold water overnight and drink in the morning and before going to sleep. Repeat this three or four days and the person will be healed.* (PL 1196 C)

This effective remedy must be prepared every night from one-half gram coarse-grained aloe and a glass of plain, cold water. The next morning the water is carefully poured in another glass without upsetting the grounds. The patient drinks half of this in the morning and the rest in the evening. The patient need not necessarily drink all the water, but the more he or she drinks the better. Aloe water looks pale yellow-green, tastes bitter, and should be drunk with little swallows. This treatment is followed three, if necessary four, days exactly as prescribed. In most cases, the threat of jaundice is then overcome (externally visible). The patient feels better, stronger, and not so tired. The yellow color fades, itching of the skin subsides, appetite returns, and the tongue is clean. The stool acquires its dark color again and the dark brown urine turns light again. From these signs one can recognize the progress of healing.

For jaundice, absolute bed rest is required, plus the sick diet which must follow a preliminary first day of strict fasting. Only when the yellow coloring of skin and eyes has disappeared should the patient get out of bed. Aloe water helps in cases of simple jaundice, but not in the rare cases when an obstructed gallstone causes a painful jaundice with fever, or when the path for the flow of bile is obstructed in some other way (as with a tumor). It cannot help in cases of gallstones and liver cancer with metastases, which lead to jaundice.

Another excellent remedy for jaundice patients is diamond water:

Whoever has jaundice should lay a diamond in wine or water, and drink the water, and this person will be cured. (PL 1262 A)

One lays a raw diamond in a water pitcher and pours water over it. All the water that the patient needs for eating and drinking should be taken from this pitcher.

Aloe water and diamond water have proved to be effective in spite of their simplicity, so that the other jaundice remedies from Hildegard medicine are usually unnecessary. This is a welcome alternative to the inadequate options offered by modern medicine for the treatment of hepatitis (infectious jaundice). Doctors are familiar neither with medicine which can combat the cause of hepatitis, nor with an effective immunization procedure to prevent its appearance.

An American study investigating gallstone operations found that half of the patients suffered from the same complaints after the operation. Gallstones, which do not cause obstruction of the bile ducts and fever, should not be removed by operation according to Hildegard. Instead the patients should let them be and learn to love them, and they will lead the persons to a sensible way of life.

Through diet and antimelancholica, the gall bladder patient can keep these attacks under control. The patient should avoid foods which are too hot, too cold, too sweet, too sour, as well as whipping cream, lard, French fries, the four kitchen poisons, beans, and coffee. With help of the blue chalcedony stone and quenched wine, anger and resentment can be neutralized, so that black bile does not flood the organism and cause trouble. (See Chapter Eleven.)

Feelings are identified by Hildegard as healing or destroying forces. For example, she urges humans not to persist in a depression. It is the responsibility of every individual to carefully choose his or her way. It is likewise the individual's responsibility if he or she chooses the wrong way by living as he or she wishes, with no sense or understanding, in complete unhappiness.

The person sits there naked like an outcast, isolated from the healthy, stripped of all good values, and with no hope of rescue. The person doesn't even turn red over his or her condition. (LVM II, 57, 58)

In this case the path to blessedness does not journey through fasting, but rather through obedience. Either a life in a monastery or a life as a hermit will help combat excesses and unhappiness.

The virtue of blessedness fights with its vice, unhappiness, which expects only tears, pain, and destruction from life. Blessedness speaks:

You don't demand a thing from God, therefore you receive nothing. You have no faith, therefore you do not receive God's help. You are downright addicted to your worries, therefore the very worst always strikes you. But I call loudly to God and receive God's help. (LVM II, 19)

Included under feelings which possess healing elements are such things as laughing, crying, singing, and dancing. About tears she writes:

Tears, which have their source in sadness, rise like bitter smoke to the eyes. They dry out the blood of a person and make the flesh grow thin. They harm a person just like spoiled food, and darken the eyes. Tears which come from joy are a milder kind. When the soul by all its tribulations remembers again that its originates from heaven and is only a wanderer on this earth, . . . then it sends gentle tears to the eyes under sighs of joy and high spirits and lets them overflow like a sweet fountain. Such tears will not harm the heart in any way, will not dry the blood, nor emaciate the flesh, and will not cause visual disturbances.
(CC 147, 23)

The goal of humankind, with its passions and emotions, is the calm composure with which one (smiling) can accept and live life. In Hildegard's beautiful language:

When the consciousness of the soul in a person perceives nothing of sadness, danger, and evil in fellow humans, then the heart of the same person opens up to joy, like flowers open toward the warmth of the sun.
(CC 149, 12)

Chapter Eleven

NERVES

QUENCHED WINE & CHALCEDONY

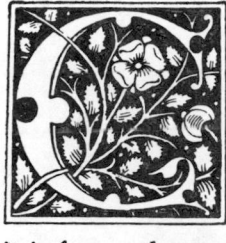an you lose your stomach or your liver? No, but you can lose your nerves! You can also lose your head or your heart, but that will not result in sickness. Yet you can lose your vision, hearing, courage, sleep, peace of mind, money, patience, and faith in God. All these things have to do with nerves. But it is funny that you can lose your nerves, and not find them again. That someone can get on my nerves and strain them seems even stranger. What funny things nerves must be!

Today, nerves are in fashion! Many people suffer from stressed nerves, depression, and anxiety, which is why there are so many tranquilizers and antidepressants on the market. Hildegard surprisingly describes how nerve disorders can be related to the soul and traced to patterns of virtues and vices (see Chapter Fifteen). Vices like anger, bitterness, or unhappiness cause the black bile in us to boil up and alter our mood.

The healing power of happiness, very important in Hildegard medicine, is effective in neutralizing black bile. Hildegard presents a variety of these important antimelancholica or "happy-makers."

1. Spelt:
daily breakfast of hot whole-grain cereal or spelt flakes.
2. Fleaseeds:
(*Psyllium*) sprinkle 1 tablespoon over food 3 times daily.
3. Pellitory:

(*Anacyclus pyrethrum*) 2-3 pinches cooked as spice.
4. Nerve Cookies:
3-5 cookies daily; see recipe below.
5. Sweet Almonds:
5-10 daily.
6. Oatmeal:
porridge.
7. Fennel:
3 times daily take fennel tablets before eating; chew fennel seeds, or drink fennel tea.
8. Savory:
(*Satureja hortensis*) 2-3 pinches cooked as spice.
9. Licorice:
(*Glycyrrhiza glabra*) 2-3 pinches cooked as spice.
10. Hyssop:
(*Hyssopus officinalis*) fresh leaves, or 2-3 pinches hyssop powder as spice cooked with chicken.
11. Quenched Wine:
see recipe below.
12. Fennel Tincture:
1-3 times daily, rub on forehead, temples, chest, and pit of the stomach or solar plexus.
13. Arum Tonic:
(*Arum maculatum*) for severe depression, 1-3 tablespoons several times daily.
14. Primrose:
(*Primula officinalis*) take a bouquet of primroses and bandage it on the heart overnight like a compress.
15. Rue:
(*Ruta graveolens*) chew one leaf after eating.
16. Chalcedony

In order to resolve anxieties, it is necessary to release them. That is why the first question in Hildegard therapy is, "Why are you here? What is troubling you?" Whatever a patient describes his or her own troubles to be, just verbalizing the symptoms helps to minimize their impact. Explaining worries cuts the worries in half! It is likewise helpful to write down concerns and thus relieve part of the burden.

It is detrimental for the nerves if persons are always reading new thrillers, or the newest bestsellers. It is far better to read the same excellent books like the Bible, so that the nerves will benefit in a marvelous way. Dale Carnegie in his wonderful book, *Don't Worry, Live,* has a fascinating collection of worries that beset individuals in all walks of life. By comparing one's own worries with those of others and observing how they coped with them, a patient can regain equilibrium and put worries in the right perspective. By reading the Bible, a patient can relate troubles and sufferings to those of God's chosen people, or to God's Son, Jesus Christ. It has a wonderful calming effect on the nerves to read such inspiring books over and over again.

Keep smiling. A smile is extremely healing as it reflects your spirit, strengthens and calms your nerves and those of other persons. A smiling face should not only be an attribute found in oriental culture, but should apply to everyone. The friendly smile on the Asian, who keeps face in all circumstances, is not only dictated by consideration for human relationships, but also fundamental to healthy soul hygiene.

With all your willpower, learn to smile in every situation. This is purely a question of will, although it is necessary to practice regularly. People cannot lose their nerves if they keep a good face even during bad times. Being thankful and glad on the inside will etch itself into the features of the face. Look in the mirror before you leave the house and smile, for, as in the words of an old favorite, "Smile, and the world smiles with you!"

Good nerves are usually a privilege of youth and depend on the graceful interplay of the five senses: clear vision, acute hearing, a fine sense of taste and smell, and a sensitive touch. Nerve cookies and the gem sardonix strengthen these faculties and slow down their aging. They also create a cheerful countenance, glad spirits and lighten a heavy heart, releasing intelligence. Here is the recipe for Hildegard's nerve or intelligence cookies.

Nerve Cookies:
1½ cups butter
3 cups brown sugar
2 eggs, well beaten
½ teaspoon salt
4 teaspoons baking powder
6 cups flour

2¼ teaspoons cinnamon
2¼ teaspoons nutmeg
½ teaspoon cloves
Cream shortening and sugar until light and fluffy. Add eggs. Combine and sift dry ingredients. Add to the creamed mixture. Knead in the last of the flour. Shape into rolls, wrap in waxed paper and chill thoroughly. When firm, slice thin, and bake at 375⁰F. Makes about 300. Add 1 cup ground or chopped almonds if desired.

Eat three to five cookies a day. They are especially beneficial for distracted school children, but do not give them too many, or they will outsmart their teacher.

In a similar way, the precious stone sardonix worn on the bare skin, and often placed in the mouth, energizes the five senses and sharpens the intellect.

This time, the best remedy has been saved for last: quenched wine. Quenched wine helps the exceptional cases of weak nerves caused by irritability, sensitiveness, or just plain anger. Fifty percent of all nerve complaints can be traced back to anger—or the anger of one's partner. Anger activates an ingredient in the blood which leads to a kind of self-poisoning. The most universal and handy remedy is quenched wine, which even helps against morning disgruntledness, weather sensitivity, and "leftovers from the night." There is not just a leftover from the day which penetrates our dream life, but also a leftover from the night which influences the whole next day. Whoever got up on that famous "wrong side of the bed"—not necessarily caused by a hangover—could not do a thing about it except wait to get through the day and hope the next day would be better. Now the day can be saved with a quenched wine. In any case it will soothe the rising anger, if used properly.

According to Hildegard, anger effects the body in a biochemical manner:

If the human soul feels that its body is menaced, then the heart, the liver, and the vessels constrict. Hereby a sort of "cloudiness" will arise from the heart [the blood becomes sour], and envelop the heart in darkness. This is how humans become sad. (CC 146, 4)

After the sadness, anger follows. When humans realize where their sadness originated, the cloud of despondency which was in their heart begins heating up all of their body fluids, especially around the bile duct where the black bile is released. This is how repressed anger silently surfaces out of the bitterness of the bile.

If one does not resist the anger, but explodes, then the bile will calm down again. Should the anger continue, however, then the smog that created the condition in the beginning will turn into a disturbing, deep, black fog. This fog then engulfs the gall bladder, releasing an extremely bitter stream (a very black bile color) into the blood. The bitter stream travels to the brain, spreading sickness and agitating the intestines and the vessels.

No other mental disturbance is as debilitating to a person as rage. In addition to this, a person will often fall into severe sicknesses, as the effects of the bile and black bile battle each other. If a person did not have the bitterness of the bile and the darkness of the black bile, then he or she would always be healthy.

In summary, Hildegard says that blood chemistry goes through a tremendous change as a result of negative influences: weather sensitivity, mood changes, and heart problems are all precipitated by sadness. One will observe two general reactions, both detrimental to health: the choleric disposition indicates explosive behavior, whereas the melancholic disposition indicates repressed anger. Repression ("that really bugs me" attitude) affects the body's weakest organs, such as the stomach (peptic ulcers), or the heart (heart attack). Repressed anger can lead to violence, which is why quenched wine is such an important catalyst in eradicating anger. It is almost like a fire extinguisher.

Hildegard offers a very fine art for regulating the cause of these disturbances:

If anyone has been provoked to anger or sadness, he or she should quickly heat up wine to boiling, then mix with a small amount of cold water. This is how the anger-causing substances are neutralized.

(CC 198, 5)

The wine can save an otherwise lost day. In addition, it prevents sleeplessness resulting from the tension of the day. We recommend the following procedure:

Take one glass of the best wine available.
Heat to boiling in a pan.
Put aside ½ glass cold water.
When bubbles surface in wine, add the cold water with one motion.

Pour back into the glass and sip. Try it once and you will never give it up. In severe situations, it is wise to prepare a thermos bottle for the day ahead. The quenched wine has less than two percent alcohol as a result of the boiling. For those sensitive to this amount, two or three tablespoons is sufficient.

Another tool of prevention is to wear the blue chalcedony stone, which aids in subduing the influences of anger:

No one who carries this stone on his skin can be put to anger, not even if the anger is justified. (PL 1258 A)

The stone is available in bracelets and necklaces, so that it can be worn next to areas that typically react to anger, such as the jugular vein and the sensitive areas of the wrist.

The teeter-totter of life has its ups and downs, its virtues and vices. Our nerves are always influenced by these opposites, especially the "bads" or the "downs." Balance or harmony between these opposites will put us back into a direct relationship with the harmony of the entire universe.

Hildegard paints the same picture in these words about the harmonies of the firmament:

By its rotation the firmament produces wonderful tones, which we cannot hear because of their very high pitch and great spaciousness, just as a mill or a wagon [wheel] has its tones when it goes around...

...the firmament can be compared to the head of a person; sun, moon, and stars are the eyes; air, the sense of hearing; the winds, the sense of smell; dew, the sense of taste; the flanks of the earth, the arms and feeling. (CC 10, 19)

Chapter Twelve

DREAMS

MESSENGERS OF THE SOUL

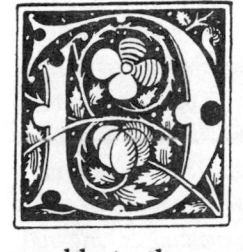 reams are as intrinsic to life as the air we breathe. An undisturbed sleep is essential to well-being. A healthy dream life rejuvenates the nerves, like a battery recharging. "As a person sleeps, the marrow within the spine regenerates." While awake, the nerves weaken and drain, comparable to the moon traveling through its phases. Similarly, plants release the life force from their roots, transmitting vital energy to blossoms in the summertime.

In like manner, the nervous system is renewed through sleep and, upon awakening, the marrow takes back the "gentle wind it sent out so that the person had his peace [during sleep]," as Hildegard would say.

Hildegard observes five different dream patterns.

1. Day Rest Dreams:
caused by unresolved problems, suppressed problems, unresolved events, and unsettled events of late evening.
2. Waking Dreams:
superficial sleep resulting from noisy disturbances, and dreams which come from eating (potato dreams).
3. Dreams Induced by Illness and precognitive dreams.
4. Prophetic Dreams:
positive, inspiring dreams experiencd by harmonious, well-balanced individuals.
5. Diabolic Dreams.

DAY REST DREAMS

Often enough, the soul when dreaming is burdened by the thoughts, opinions, and emotions that preoccupy the mind while awake. The soul will be affected by these elements in dream life to such an extent that it becomes as bloated as rising sourdough, regardless whether the thoughts are good or bad.

. . . If a person goes to sleep mentally occupied with unfitting joy or sadness, with wrath or fear, with lust for power or the like, the devil in deviousness will play upon these vulnerabilities. When a person falls asleep with lusty thoughts of the flesh, the devil's mockery holds these thoughts up to him once more by showing him living figures of those with whom he has had sexual relations. These can be the living bodies of the dead, even if he had never regarded them with the eyes of the flesh. It seems to the dreamer that he is awake and the dead are still living, that he enjoys the pleasures of sinful lust and ejaculation. Even the dreamer's semen is degraded by the devil's mockery. Just as the devil plays his deceitful game with the waking individual, he does not leave him in peace in his sleep. Just as the air in the water drives the millwheel and mills the grain, the soul incites the body of the sleeping and waking individual to all sorts of deeds. (CC 82, 33, ff)

Often a confused and preoccupied mind prevents one from falling asleep. The accompanying sorrow, fear, anxiety, and other contradictory emotions disturb the blood chemistry. The vessels constrict and dilate, unable to relax sufficently for sleep. When anything of a positive nature that evokes happiness is seen, heard, or felt, the blood vessels will relax to experience the joy. Yet even these relaxed vessels may not induce the necessary sleep, unless the overall temperament is in order. Restlessness and sleeplessness will recur until at last peace is found with the emotions.

WAKING DREAMS

But when noise and turmoil or loud conversation prevail in the surroundings of a sleeping person, the air will echo. Then the outside air will strike back the air which is found in the person, because the elements are also present in the human body. As soon as the soul notices this movement in the air, it will draw its energy back to itself and cause the person to wake up. It often happens that someone unwillingly awakens through sudden noise, touch, or unexpectedly in some other way.

(CC 85, 14)

Those awakened by noise disturbances, such as a baby crying, a snoring spouse, or a barking dog, suffer a deprived dream life, and since they have little dreaming, there is no rest. Those who wake up after a harmonious dream cycle will enjoy a completely rejuvenated nervous system. This has been confirmed by dream researchers. The nightly fluctuation of periodic awakening is accepted today as healthy and refreshing. The leadened deep sleep in one stretch will not create a refreshed awakening. The refreshed morning arising is related to dreaming, whether the dreams are remembered or not.

As soon as the marrow of the sleeper increases and is strengthened, the soul restores the whole continuity of the sleeping body. In this manner it takes back the gentle wind, which had been sent out of the marrow of the individual for his repose, and the person awakes again. If one often awakens at intervals and between times falls asleep unexpectedly, then the marrow will not acquire its complete richness and energy, and the limbs will not be completely rested. But the person who often wakes up and then sleeps again will invigorate marrow and limbs in a very pleasant manner. It is similar to the baby who often sucks and again stops sucking to gather strength for its recuperation. (CC 84, 31)

DREAMS INDUCED BY ILLNESS

It frequently happens that a person sleeping on a side or some other part of the body becomes uncomfortable or irritated, or suffers some bodily discomfort. Because the individual is sensitive, his or her soul sees and feels these annoyances and senses that the body coupled with it could be injured. It gathers its strength, draws in the wind it send forth from the marrow, and in this way awakens the individual from its sleep.

(CC 85, 7)

Older people with cardiac disorders may often wake up hyperventilating with a fluttering heart after a nightmare. Nightmares and sleeplessness seem to be the fate of modern humanity. Modern treatment for such cases includes sleeping pills, tranquilizers, or psychotherapy, all more-or-less useless. But an excellent remedy is wood betony leaves, to be used in a little herb pillow placed next to the skin during the night.

89

HILDEGARD'S MEDICINE

Wood betony leaves (*Stachys officinalis*) should only be used for herb pillows, never drunk as tea. Health stores have dried wood betony leaves, which are best sewn into a pillow. A pound of leaves is stuffed into an old stocking and knotted at both ends. Over that one can pull a pillow case made out of sheer gauze cloth. Through the scent, and perhaps through the fine dust which settles on the skin of the dreamer, unpleasant dreams stop immediately.

Whoever is plagued by wrong dreams should have betony leaves close by when going to sleep, and this person will see and feel fewer bad dreams.   (PL 1182 B - 1183 A)

PROPHETIC DREAMS

When God let sleep descend on Adam, his soul saw in a truly prophetic fashion many things, because it was still free from sin. In like manner, the soul of a sleeping person can also see many things prophetically, if that same person is not burdened by sins.   (CC 82, 22)

Those light, joyous individuals like Adam and Eve and Jacob, who are not weighted down by sins and vices, will receive heavenly messages and experience prophetic dreams. Such persons are of an extraordinary nature, full of grace and peaceful in character. They seldom have nightmares and more often have enlightening dreams of prophecy. Like Adam's brothers, it is possible for all of us to receive heavenly messages and experience prophetic dreams.

Because the human soul is of God, it sometimes sees the truth and the future while the body sleeps. It knows what awaits us and sometimes it knows what happens. . .When thoughts are positive and holy, the grace of God reveals truth to the dreamer.   (CC 82, 28)

DIABOLIC DREAMS

The soul is often weakened by the devil's antics, or disturbed by the darkening of the spirit. Thus the soul loses its clear vision and suffers delusions of the imagination. Negative thoughts entice the devil's influence to such a degree as to terrorize the soul. The devil will insidiously undermine human thought with delusions and lies. Even saints and holy people may perceive shameful visions, mesmerized by Satan's sinister laughter.   (CC 82, 32)

90

Diabolic dreams and nightmares can be easily remedied and positively controlled with the aid of the pillow filled with wood betony leaves (see above).

Besides the betony herb pillow, Hildegard suggests the precious stone, jasper, to regulate one's dream-life. Thunder and lightening dreams may announce threatening sicknesses and may even cause sicknesses. Persons with such dreams should take a jasper to bed with them for a longer period of time. The cold jasper placed on the skin is helpful, "because then the fantastic forms and fiends will fly away and get lost."(PL 1257 B)

In all cases, a natural biological sleep is essential. For all of those who rely on sleeping pills and other drugs, their sleep is not sleep at all. Rather it is anesthesia which severely inhibits the natural dreaming phases and the fluctuating patterns of natural sleep. For these people, we recommend sauna treatments while inhaling chestnut extract. This technique evokes relaxation, while the chestnut cleanses the brain. An aid for those who still have difficulty sleeping is one cup hot wine with one tablespoon valerian root.

Just as the sun is the light of the day, so is the soul the light of the body awake. And just as the moon is the light of the night, so also is the soul the light of the body asleep. Whenever the body of a sleeping person has the right warmth, its marrow will be warmed in the right proportion and degree. When the person is free from the storm of conflict and moral contradictions, he or she will very often see the truth, because then the knowledge of the soul is at rest. The moon shines its light bright and clear, whenever the night is free from the turbulence of clouds and winds. But when a storm of various and contrary thoughts controls the body and spirit of the person awake, and he or she goes to sleep with this storm, then that which the soul sees in dreams is almost always false. The knowledge of the soul is so darkened under such contradictions, that it cannot see the truth. The moon cannot shine clearly in a storm of clouds. (CC 83, 27 ff)

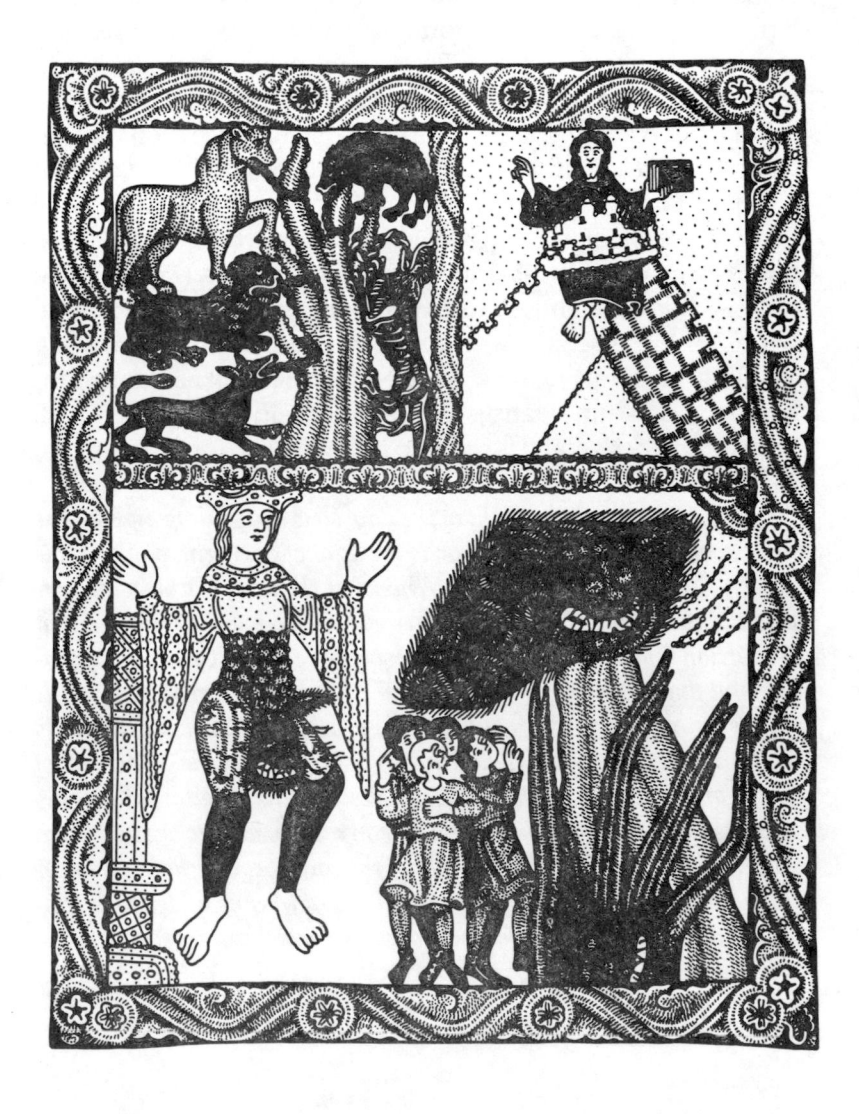

Chapter Thirteen

RHEUMATISM
CURES WITH
GOLD & QUINCE

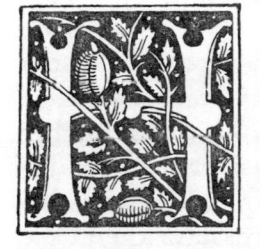 ildegard sees the basic roots of all kinds of rheumatism and gout as being directly connected with the struggle for life, with fear, or with a disturbance of the metabolism through overeating and drinking. About fever and the critical days:

Whenever a person suffers from various troubles, fear, and the result of many different foods and drinks, so that through these unsuitable foods and drinks different and harmful juices and mucus [livores] collect, then the upset and tired soul will break down, plagued by unpleasantness, and will give up its life energy to a certain degree. (CC 163, 11)

Hildegard says that a harmonious interaction of all the bodily functions continually restores the organism's unimpeded function. The secretion of the hormonal glands, the function of the organs, the chemistry of the tissues and the body fluids, are all an intricate part of the total organism and influence our emotions and overall integrity, just as they affect our spirituality and vice-versa.

Sometimes harmful body fluids produce a smoke in a person [gas together with blood] which rises to the brain and poisons it so badly that it becomes foolish, forgetful, and abandoned of all its senses.

(CC 145, 8)

From her visionary point of view 800 years ago, Hildegard offers a real concept of healing. She describes the root causes of disease, employing at the same time a style which makes for simplicity and understanding. She recognizes that the vitality of the whole body must be restored in order to heal and repair. The word "rheumatism" did not exist in Hildegard's day: instead she calls it *paralyse*, or sometimes *gutta* (gout), which one can translate as being lame.

Persons with soft tissues and porous flesh, who overindulge in heavy wine, will often be plagued with gout. Due to excessive drinking, the secretion of harmful body fluids increases in people with soft flesh and will suddenly attack one of their joints and destroy it, as if with burning arrows, or like massive floods which can destroy a mill or other structure. The fluids would likewise destroy the joints if the grace of God and the life energy within did not prevent it. Nevertheless, they kill and destroy some joints and make them useless. (CC 161, 28)

Millions of patients suffer their worst pain from the attacks of rheumatism which medical science has not yet been able to cure. The general term "rheumatic affliction" covers a number of more or less serious, painful, treatment-resistant, chronic disorders such as rheumatoid arthritis, gout, and lumbago with inflammation of the joints, nerves, and soft tissues. Rheumatic afflictions also include neuralgia, which generally arises from a disorder of adjoining parts of the body like ligaments, bones, and joints causing rheumatic back pain and sciatica, a neuralgia of the sciatic nerve.

With the help of Hildegard's cure, the pain and agony of this difficult disease can be prevented in the early stages and relieved in the more advanced stages. In the final stages, it can at least be relieved by changing the life style, using positive thinking, applying the Hildegard diet, and by intensive cleansing of body and soul.

Many patients have gone from one physician to another in a fruitless quest for the cure of their pain and agony. The present-day approach with painkillers and anti-inflammatories like cortisone, indomethacins, or aspirin, as employed in modern medicine for this disease, is of no value. Conventional medicine cannot eliminate causative factors in order to overcome systemic disturbances merely by suppressing pain and symptoms, and failing to correct the underlying causes.

Most people taking painkillers will not change their familiar

life style, because they are under the impression that these remedies possess specific curative properties. The recurrent pains,
which grow more severe with time, require more and stronger
painkillers. Modern painkillers have proven their ineffectiveness
as far as permanent benefit is concerned, and actually add to the
damage. There is no question that a drug may provide relief of
pain, but at what a price! Use over a long period of time may
even undermine the body's immune system and suppress the
acute symptoms of the disease, which may then move from an
active rheumatic condition into a chronic state.

Suppressive measures destroy the reactive powers of the
body, like pain, and lead to a more chronic condition. All acute
symptoms are reactions on the part of the body in its endeavor
to rid itself of toxins and overcome an abnormal condition. These
acute processes must not be suppressed. Measures that suppress the body's reactive processes are not only not helpful, but
actually cause harm, converting a simple disease into its more
advanced chronic state with further damage.

Although focal infection has been considered to be a cause
of rheumatoid arthritis, the extirpation of tonsils, gall bladder,
appendix, ovaries, uterus, and the other so-called "foci of infection," the indiscriminate extraction of teeth, and repeated drainage of the sinuses are definitely harmful in the long run. Surgery
may provide immediate relief, but it increases damage and fails
to correct the underlying causes. The indiscriminate removal of
organs or tissues, in the hope that this will correct the condition,
has proven a costly delusion. The need is not for surgery or
antibiotics that destroy bacteria, but for the application of measures that rebuild the organism and restore normal organ
function.

The tonsils, for example, are lymphatic glands and serve to
eliminate toxins from the system. They become inflamed when
the lymphatic system is overburdened with work. Surgery does
not rebuild better lymphatic drainage. The important thing is to
restore lymphatic drainage to a normal condition. This is readily accomplished with the elimination of the causative factors
and with Hildegard's remedy—horehound soup (see Chapter
Four). In addition, special care should be taken to promote the

elimination of toxins by way of the kidneys, skin, lungs, and intestines. Only when the underlying causes are corrected, and the source of the trouble overcome, is real improvement possible.

From the time of Hildegard until the eighteenth century, the word "rheumatism" was unknown and was translated as "catarrh." Using her own language, she describes over 100 rheumatism remedies, together with the clinical pictures which rheumatics observe to some extent in themselves. Mostly she writes about gout, a poisoning or contamination of the body, which literally translated means flooding, disintegrating, falling to pieces, or in Latin, *paralyse*.

So-called "rheumatism," the large family of rheumatic complaints, belongs to this *paralyse* group. It involves torturing pains in joints, muscles, nerves, tendons, and vertebrae, which either swell, inflame, crack, or sprain. In agreement with today's scientific findings, Hildegard describes rheumatism as a disturbance in the metabolism of the supportive tissues, resulting from a bad mixture of body fluids (dyskrasie). The concept dyskrasie is modern and of immediate interest because of present-day information about metabolism, immunity, inner hormone secretion, and allergies.

If the basal metabolism is upset [humores] through sicknesses, or sickness-making and unhealthy nutrition, the fluids themselves will drive and push the undigested foods and drinks back out . . . If the bad fluids increase, they will cause a foggy smoke in the whole person [foul, intestinal gas]. This spreads in the bowels, in the stomach, and in the whole body and releases all the remaining serious sicknesses [pestes] in mankind. (CC 151, 25)

Hildegard traces the diseases of the rheumatic family directly to a fundamental disturbance of the four world elements on a personal and cosmic order, as a result of a detrimental life style. She especially warns us against the personal psychic risk factors (vices), which are detrimental to health, because disturbances of the cosmic order can cause the 24 basic diseases of man.

In much the same way as the elements hold the world together, they also provide for continuity in the human body. Just as the elements and their effects are spread throughout the entire world, they distribute themselves and their duties in human beings in such a way that the human individual is continually sustained by the elements. Fire, air, water, and earth are in human beings. Human beings consist of these elements. They have warmth from fire, breath from air, blood from water, and flesh from earth. In the same way, fire is responsible for the sight of the human individual, air for hearing, water for movement, and earth for gait.

When the elements are properly ordered in the human being, they sustain and make this person well. However, should they fail to harmonize in this person, they make the person ill and kill him or her. Mixtures of humors drawn from warmth, moisture, blood, and flesh are present in the human being. When these humors remain tranquilly active in the proper relationship, a healthy human being is the natural result. When, on the other hand, they assail an individual too much, they weaken and kill this person. (CC 49, 29)

One of the 24 basic diseases caused by the discord of the four elements is a form of arthritis where the "spine is totally contracted [*spondilitis deformans*, Still's disease and Bechterefft's disease], but he will live a long life, until his sufferings are over." (CC 52, 20)

By far, the most patients suffer from arthritis which affects one or more joints of the body and can lead to terrible pain. It occurs in many forms. Arthritis deformans is a sign of aging in middle-aged and older people (the hypertropic type). Rheumatoid arthritis, also known as atrophic arthritis, starts with inflammation and then leads to a wasting or degeneration of the tissues. It mostly occurs in younger people. Infectious arthritis results from tubercular gonorrhea, streptococci, other bacteria or toxins. Spondilitis deformans is a form of arthritis where the spine is ankylosed or stiffened. Polyarthritis affects many joints. Soft-tissue rheumatism, or muscular rheumatism, includes lumbago (lower back), and myalgia. Rheumatic inflammation of nerves (neuritis, neuralgia such as sciatic rheumatism) finishes up the long list.

Another form of arthritis caused by the four elements is a development of cerebral arteriosclerosis, the most frequent cause of a brain infarct, resulting in the clinical picture of a stroke. Hildegard describes very precisely this cerebrovascular disease, which begins with cracking and buzzing in the ears and which may lead to paralysis.

They [the four elements] produce a dangerous-sounding tone and the sound of thunder. And this tone sounds all the way to the veins, to the marrow of the bones, and to the temples. Whoever suffers from this will become lame and lose strength all over the body. (CC 52, 35)

Patients with arthritis where one or more joints are inflamed, as in polyarthritis, have intense pain.

Persons with an unstable metabolism and constantly changing reactions in the management of body warmth, cold, or moisture will be blown like air in the body, back and forth, and will be plagued by paralysis. (CC 162, 35)

Hildegard describes how critical conditions come about through fever and infections, because the person's digestive organs are overworked and unable to digest food properly. The result is an increase of poisons and waste products. When the excretory organs such as skin, kidneys, liver, lungs, and intestines are exhausted, far too many toxins accumulate in the entire organism. The body becomes lazy and tired due to overfeeding and a lack of exercise. An excess of fats and proteins clogs the arteries and inside walls of the colon, where food is absorbed.

The accumulation of morbid matter can block the intake of essential nutrients. Morbid bacteria created by rotten, undigested food create wind and foul gas in the intestine, and pass through the entire organism and weaken the body. Metabolism is impaired, circulation slowed down, and a tremendous amount of life energy is lost.

Through this vicious circle persons feel tired, down-hearted, and they freeze all over.

In this way the harmful body juices [noxi humores] start moving and fever increases, because the soul has given up its rule of life. Then even the amount of blood in a person decreases and the intestines and other organs dry up. Warmth, which is necessary for liver and other inner organs, passes on to the skin, while coldness remains in the body. The soul lies there distressed and waits in despair, wondering whether it should leave the body. Thus it waits mostly until the seventh day, because it cannot free itself any earlier from the body fluids and slimes. But as soon as it notices that the storm of juices subsides through the grace of God, it will gather all its energy and drive those fluids and slimes back out of the body through sweating. In this way, the person regains health. (CC 163, 17 ff)

Arthritis is deadly, unless the style of life is dramatically changed. The old habitual ways of eating and drinking overtax the entire organism. A reckless and irresponsible way of living with no consideration for oneself will slowly cause a loss of energy and certain death.

When the soul is burdened to such a degreee with harmful liquids and slimes [waste products], so that it cannot drive them out of the body, and when it notices that the grace of God is no longer standing at one's side, it will submit to God's decision and leave the body. (CC 164, 8 ff)

True gout is described by Hildegard as "gutta" or dropsy, a special form of rheumatism. This, too, is caused by a disturbance in metabolism, whereby uric acid settles in deposits in the joints, particularly in foot and finger joints, and causes violent attacks. The clinical picture for gout, according to Hildegard, is already in the introduction, but she describes it more thoroughly in her diagnostic:

Whoever has soft, voluptuous flesh in the body and often consumes all kinds of tasty delicacies, will be easily attacked by gout of the big toe. . . It also happens with persons who eat many different things in confusion, so that they easily become sick. Whenever such persons over-indulge in all these tasty delicacies, then the bad body juices increase, overflow, and multiply so much that it is impossible to restrain them. They flow back and forth out of order and finally fall down into the lower body extremities where they rage and storm in the legs and feet. And because they find no exit and want to move upward again but cannot, they end up remaining in the lower extremities where they are changed into slime [waste] and burden. Such a person feels the gout in the legs and feet and suffers great pains, so that the person can hardly walk any more. (CC 101, 20 ff)

It is interesting that women seldom suffer from gout, since the excess bad body juices are removed through menstruation.

HOW CAN ARTHRITIS BE DETECTED IN TIME & PREVENTED?

Arthritis takes years before one becomes aware of its serious

99

nature. None of the early symptoms should be overlooked if the more advanced form is to be avoided. Pain or discomfort in the joints is an early symptom. A feeling of numbness or stiffness, an aching or sore back, as well as cold clammy hands and feet, are all warning signals.

The frequent common cold is also a forerunner of rheumatic disease, weakening the body and its resistance. It is an established fact with Hildegard that the chronic cold, with its runny nose and bronchial cartarrh, cannot be cured until the weaknesses in stomach and digestion have been eliminated:

Those who have a cold weak stomach and weak intestines [gastritis and bad digestion] send a cold moist smoke [gas] into their brain, which is discharged like a cooked poison through nose and mouth.

(CC 132, 6)

The brain uses the sense organs as permanent cleansing outlets. Hildegard describes how the brain cleans itself through eyes, ears, nose, and mouth. These are its windows which are opened for fresh air and moisture. The cold and wet filth from bad juices are gathered in the nose and throat and ejected out of the body with a blast of air. If this cleansing is suppressed, the person can lose his or her senses and dry out. The stomach and brain cannot tolerate the rotting waste products, and must throw them out, just as the ocean throws out its filth and rubbish. (CC 132, 10)

Since a runny nose has a cleansing function, it should not be suppressed or obstructed, or severe rheumatic ailments may follow. Hildegard even describes how mucus can be caused through exotic and unusual cooking. Different exquisite kinds of cheese may cause mucus which, however, one can prevent through the use of cumin as the universal cheese spice. "Smelling herbs" help expel excess mucus.

If a person once enjoys a new unfamiliar meal, or drinks new strange wine or other unusual drink, then the other harmful juices within will be agitated by these foreign juices and, through cleansing, run back out of the nose. . .

If a person would in some way suppress or prevent such a cleansing, he or she would be harmed in the same way as if this person would retain stool or urine, so that they cannot exit on time. But if the foreign

juices add to the existing juices to such an extent that a severe pain dev-
lops, then one must use smelling herbs, so that the juices flow out more
easily. (CC 134, 19 ff)
(For more information, see Chapter Four.)

Arthritis can be caused by faulty digestion, overeating and
bad nutrition. The four seasonal poisons, strawberries, peaches,
plums, and leeks, produce harmful body fluids, the so-called
mali humores. Combine this with a disorderly life style and dis-
content, or the tendency towards negative emotions, feelings,
and thoughts, and life can be killed. Fortunately, correction is
possible through healthful living, together with various forms
of physiotherapy treatment.

Cleansing (purging) is an art in itself, according to Hildegard. An age-old motto, *"qui bene purgat, bene curat,"* is still
valid for today: "Who purges well, cures well." Hildegard recommends purge pills from mild medicinal plants, which remove
excess harmful waste products, especially mucus from the nose
and throat. Used together with bloodletting, pain and inflammation in the head, chest, and stomach area will disappear. Purge
pills clear away only the harmful bad juices and retain the good
ones. When the first symptoms of these arthritis-causing waste
products appear, and so that the disease develops no further,
eight purge pills should be taken every morning before breakfast
for ten days. Each pill is dipped in honey because of its bitterness. Stomach and abdomen should be kept warm in bed with
a sheep skin or badger fur (see page 106). After taking the pills,
the patient should go for a walk until he or she feels the relaxing
effect. At noon, the patient should eat a cream of spelt soup, or
a chicken broth with spelt dumplings. The purge pills have
proved successful for sicknesses with severe mucous obstruction
or hyper-salivation.

Hildegard warns emphatically against laxatives which can
cause serious heart damage. Especially rheumatic persons
should beware of laxatives, which are used much too much
today.

Laxatives, which clean the stomach, are of no use for persons who
are very sick and in such bad shape that they become lame [paralyzed]
from them. They are also useless for such persons who have an overly

101

*flexible body juice metabolism, . . . because the so-conditioned juices flow
more quickly after their digestion through the stomach, back and forth
between skin and flesh, as well as in the vessels, and are not to be found
at the same time in the stomach. If a laxative comes into the stomach,
it will find no juice there at all for cleansing.* (CC 135, 10)

No one better than Hildegard knows so exactly the processes
of metabolism. She mentions a purging cookie, the so-called
"ginger-cleansing cookie," with which only the harmful juices
leave the organism and the good juices are retained.

*Persons who are worn down from a gouty paralysis and are plagued
by the aforementioned juices, should use to their advantage the powder
from precious and good medicinal herbs [to prepare cookies], because the
good and pleasant smell of valuable spices subdues, controls, and
weakens through its mild effect the harmful smoke [noxi humores],
which originates from the above mentioned juices and stimulates the bad
juices [mali humores].* (CC 135, 22)

With the ginger-cleansing cookie one can begin a Hildegard
fasting cure, and prevent and treat rheumatism. It is a gentle substitute for unpleasant Glauber's salt, which is hard on the heart.
This universal remedy preserves health and prevents sickness
by cleansing the whole metabolic system. Fatty juices containing
waste, poisons (*limus*) and decaying metabolic products (feces),
as well as decomposing waste products (*tabes*), are washed out
of the body.

THE COMPLETE
HILDEGARD ARTHRITIS TREATMENT

The complete Hildegard arthritis treatment involves the
complete person, since arthritis is not a local process, but rather
a general disease with a general feeling of sickness and a disturbed basal metabolism. Circulation and digestion are poor,
hormone regulation impaired and possibilities of regeneration
lacking. In order to put an arthritic patient who has "come apart"
back together again, radical measures must be taken in order to
eliminate all provoking causes on a long-term basis. Even in the
most advanced cases, the complete Hildegard arthritis treatment
seems to be the only therapy which can help in the long run.

To heal arthritis successfully one must detoxify, purify and regenerate the whole organism. Patients, and those doing the treating, must be very conscientious and have perseverance and patience. Because the arthritic patient suffers from a lack of energy, Hildegard recommends bringing the *viriditas* (life energy) into action, which is found in the healing elements throughout the whole cosmos. Only measures that aid in the elimination of toxins, improve circulation, rebuild vitality, and promote normal functioning are of help.

The complete Hildegard arthritis treatment, depicted by the six age-old golden rules of life, can give back to the arthritic patient the harmony he or she has lost. New life energy pours out of:

1. The healing forces from the four elements: fire, air, water, and earth.
2. The curative value found in proper food and drink.
3. The power of life itself through exercise and rest.
4. The restoration of health through sleeping and waking.
5. Regeneration through elimination and secretion.
6. The healing force found in the Christian virtues.

Hildegard sees health in a direct relationship with the order of the four earth elements in the complete (macro) cosmos and in humankind, the micro cosmos. Through this relationship or balance, the vital living functions are maintained:

As has been described many times, the elements supply, just like they hold the whole world together, in the same way also the structure for the human body. Their extension and function are so distributed in the whole person, that the person is kept going continually through them, just like the elements are spread throughout the rest of the world and are active. In humans are fire, air, water, and earth, and they are made out of them. From fire, humans have [body] warmth; from air, breath; from water, blood; and from the earth, body. Humans can thank fire for seeing, air for hearing, water for movement, and earth for walking. (CC 49, 29)

As is commonly known today, human ignorance of the cosmic laws has catastrophic consequences, not only for the cosmos, but also for humanity's personal life. The modern brutal destruction of creation through technology is an example of humanity's disregard for the four world elements. Likewise respect for the cosmic laws recognizes the healing forces in the four world elements and employs them effectively.

All Hildegard remedies possess their effectiveness through these healing forces and preserve health as well as prevent sickness, especially chronic illness. The universal remedies are many-sided; depending on one's predisposition, they can be used once a year as a course of treatment. Naturally their simple and reliable prescriptions are with no harmful side-effects—as always with Hildegard's remedies.

The famous spring tonic with vermouth elixir is Hildegard's most effective remedy for preventing all serious chronic illnesses such as rheumatism, tendency towards flu and colds, arteriosclerosis, coronary illnesses, diabetes, and strokes. Vermouth stimulates the complete immune system of the body and provides a good kidney function. In this manner, poisons and waste products from blood vessels and supportive tissues are thoroughly cleared away and eliminated. Even arteriosclerotic plaques (surplus of fats and proteins) clogging the vessels, or causing stones in the gall bladder or kidney, are removed and discharged. Bitter vermouth stimulates the circulation of the stomach, which is important because it facilitates the digestion of food. Vermouth elixir is described in detail in Chapter Six.

The Hildegard gold cure consists of gold paste and gold cookies, which are prepared from fine nugget gold powder, spelt or wheat flour, and water. Two original packages of pure nugget gold powder (not synthetic gold from coins or gold bars) are required. On the first day, a gold paste is prepared from six-tenths of a gram of gold, one tablespoon of (spelt) flour, and one teaspoon of water, and is eaten one-half hour before breakfast. On the second day, the gold paste, prepared as before, is baked, and this gold cookie eaten likewise one-half hour before breakfast. This cure suffices for a whole year. [Editor's Note: Large amounts of gold may be toxic if taken internally.]

The gold cure is a universal prophylactic and therapeutic remedy for arthritis and gout as well as for stomach ctarrh and flu susceptibility, the first pre-symptoms for arthritis. The gold cure also prevents colds, and illnesses caused by colds, which can lead to dangerous sicknesses in elderly persons. It has always been a wish of famous doctors to find a universal remedy which could strengthen people's power of resistance in order to heal sicknesses and maintain health. We know today that the greatest part of the immune system is located in the lymphatic glands all along the intestinal tract. The finest gold dust does not dissolve and therefore stimulates and strengthens the immune system via the mucous linings of the intestines.

In this sense, the Hildegard gold cure is one of the best contributions in the struggle against civilization's sicknesses like rheumatism or perhaps even AIDS, or other serious viral illnesses, which may yet afflict human beings in the future.

Gold is warm and has the nature of the sun and is almost like the element air. If someone is rheumatic, this person should take gold, cook it so that no more dirt is present, but also so that nothing gets lost, and then grind it to powder. Then this person should take a little fine flour, about half of a handful, and knead it with water. To this dough add from the gold powder an amount of six-tenths of a gram and eat it early in the morning before breakfast on the first day. In the same manner, the person proceeds on the second day, except that he or she should make cookies with the flour and gold powder, and eat them on this second day before breakfast. Gold prepared and eaten in this way will take away arthritis [gout] for a year. The gold remains for two months in the stomach, but does not attack the mucous membrane, nor make it ulcerous. Rather it warms and cleans it without endangering the stomach, if the person has a cold or is suffering from phlegm. If a healthy person does this, health will be preserved, and if a sick person does this, he or she will get healthy. (PL 1347 A/C)

All forms of arthritis with severe pain, such as shoulder, elbow, and finger arthritis, can be treated with Hildegard's arthritic ointment. The ointment, formulated from vermouth and deer fat, is rubbed on the afflicted area in front of an elm wood fire. Pain is relieved and the regenerative power of the cartilage activated. Hildegard describes the effective arthritic ointment:

Squeeze vermouth and take four parts of this juice, two parts of deer fat and two parts of deer marrow, and mix into a salve. Whoever suffers seriously from rheumatism, so that the joints almost break, should mas-

105

sage the salve where it hurts, in front of a fire, and this person will get
well again. (PL 1173 B)

And whoever is plagued by rheumatism should light an elm wood
fire, be warmed immediately by the fire, and the rheumatism will depart
in that same hour. (PL 1242 A)

Who would ever have thought that the fragrant golden quinces, which ripen every fall in gardens, can so thoroughly purge and decontaminate the body, so that the healthy person never gets arthritis and the arthritic person is healed? Eating quinces often is one of the best preventatives against all forms of rheumatism.

Eaten raw, the golden quince fruit harms neither sick nor healthy.
But cooked or baked it is very beneficial for sick and healthy persons. The
arthritic person should often eat this fruit cooked and baked, and it will
destroy in this person the rheumatic toxins, so that they can neither dull
the senses [cerebral sclerosis], nor break the limbs [arthrose deformans],
nor leave the person helpless. (PL 1220 C)

Every Hildegard patient should enjoy a quince cure in the fall. Quince can be cooked for twenty minutes in water or wine, or baked like apples in a cake or pie. Quince marmalade, jelly and candy, in which almonds and galgant can be mixed, are tasty ways to enjoy this fruit.

The most potent pain reliever is rheumatic powder, or celery seed powder, which has a carminative, spasmolytic, and soothing effect. Together with celery seed, the remedy contains such spices as rue, cloves, and saxifrage. One to three teaspoons should be taken before breakfast and chewed slowly. If it tastes too strong, celery powder can be sprinkled on bread with quince jelly.

Whoever is plagued by gout, so that the mouth is distorted and the
limbs tremble [Parkinson's] and is pulled together in the limbs [arthrose
deformans], should powder celery seeds and add one-third of that
amount of rue to it, and a bit less nutmeg powder than rue, and less
cloves than nutmeg, and less saxifrage than cloves. Make a powder out
of these ingredients and gout will go away, because this is the best
remedy against gout. (PL 1139 D)

Badger furs in many forms are recommended for various aches and pains. Back pains can be alleviated by sleeping on a badger fur in bed. Badger shoes or inner soles guarantee warm feet. Badger belts or vests can also help arthritic pains by providing heat.

Great strength is in the badger fur. Make a belt out of it and put it on the naked skin and all sickness . . . in you will cease, as if a great storm ends with good weather and a good calm breeze. No dangerous sickness will attack you.

. . . . But make shoes and boots out of the badger fur also and put them on and you will have healthy legs and feet. (PL 1333 A)

My first experience with badger slippers came from an 85-year-old lady, who called me shortly before a foot amputation. Her toes were blue and cold and the doctor found no pulse any more. This is a routine case like many others with elderly diabetic patients. After walking in badger slippers for a few hours, her blood circulation was so improved that the amputation was no longer necessary.

For soft tissue and nerve rheumatism, the curled mint tonic can bring relief. It is excellent for neuralgic pains, rheumatic, back and sciatic pains, or if it hurts all over. Even neuralgia which may arise from irritation or injury to various nerves, or pain due to exposure to cold, can be helped by curled mint tonic. For lasting results, the removal of underlying causes is necessary in addition to the tonic.

And whoever is plagued by gout [arthritis] should pulverize curled mint and sieve the juice. Add some wine to it and drink this tonic mornings, evenings, and at bedtime, and the gout will recede. (PL 1161 D)

The curled mint tonic, one of the strongest painkillers in Hildegard medicine, is taken three times a day in a tiny sherry glass.

Fasting followed by the Hildegard diet is the best protection against arthritis. Because overeating is one of the causes of arthritis, fasting and a complete switch to new eating habits, based on spelt and spelt products, can restore health. Most people think that to rebuild health the eating of large quantities of food is necessary. But it is not the food we eat, but the food we digest and assimilate that nourishes the body. Eating beyond the digestive capacity overtaxes the digestive organs, increases fatigue, decreases life energy, and adds to the toxins in the body. The arthritic patient must discard all harmful foods and subsist on a diet of natural, easily digestible foods. (For more information, see Chapter Eight).

Hildegard recommends, especially for persons suffering from weak tendons and joints with symptoms of wear, a restorative soup made out of knuckle of veal. This soup contains easily digestible cartilage, which stimulates the growing of new cartilage due to bio-available calcium. Knuckles of veal are cooked in two to three quarts of water for several hours to obtain a nourishing broth. Seasoned with herbs and cream of spelt and eaten several times a week, this soup is a basic cure to rebuild cartilage tissue and strengthen supportive tissues.

Not every water is beneficial. Some water which contains too many salts can damage and burden the body and especially the supportive tissues. An arthritic person should only drink water which is able to remove waste products from the body. Hildegard suggests saline spring and river water from eastern areas, which originates in various parts of the Earth. It is pure and somewhat green in color and has its source in sandy ground.

If an arthritic patient drinks this water often, this person will receive health back, because it takes away the harmful vapor, the rottenness and the bad juices [mali humores] like a good salve. (CC 24, 16 ff)

Exercise and rest must be done in moderation, for an excess or deficiency of one or the other may have an injurious effect. Adequate rest, often essential for arthritic persons, can easily be overdone, and too much may lead to further atrophy of the tissues and cause more extensive crippling. Strenuous exercise, taking walks that are too long, and overactivity or forced activity may result in more fatigue with further inflammation and damage to the afflicted joints. Exercise without strain is excellent, such as swimming, bicycling, or just simply sitting on a table and letting the legs swing back and forth. Appropriate arthritis gymnastics or meditative dance, autogenous training, or yoga, combined with correct breathing technique, offer far-reaching elements of healing.

How often do people find that they are extremely tired even after a full night's sleep? This is due to the fact that even after sleep their nerves are still in tension. We lose our life energy, if we are under stress or tension, full of fear or panic. Hatred greed, jealousy, and unhappiness also add to the dissipation of energy. Mere sleep or physical rest is not enough to counteract these debilitating influences. (To learn more about natural sleep and its rehabilitating powers for nerves and health, refer to Chapter Twelve.)

Most people are searching for complex, mysterous remedies, but Hildegard proposes very simple measures. A hot bath, utilizing the healing forces of water, will improve circulation and promote better elimination. Following the hot bath, the person should slip into a bathrobe without drying and retire with a hot water bottle on the feet. Regular sun baths whenever possible are very helpful, although caution is needed, as the hottest rays of the sun (at noon) are weakening. Habits that are injurious to health like smoking, alcohol, late hours, and excesses of all kinds must be eliminated. Bad shoes, tight clothing, anything that impairs or weakens circulation must be eliminated.

Using the four elements and their healing forces helps restore the function of the elimination organs and provides better health. Fresh air, deep breathing, and appropriate exercise help the lungs eliminate. Hildgard's diet, emphasizing simple non-irritating food, corrects intestinal sluggishness. Hot baths and rest are helpful for the kidneys. Sauna and dry brushing promotes sweating, so that the skin can eliminate better. The king of all remedies, fasting, provides a much-needed rest for the overworked digestive organs, and assists in an adequate elimination of toxins which have accumulated in the system.

When treatment with natural methods begins, suppressive or stimulative measures are immediately discontinued and the body starts to clean house. Poisons from the deepest nooks and crevices must be cleaned out. The body cleans house in many ways, not only primarily through the bowels, but through all the organs of elimination: the lungs, kidneys, and skin. Fever, for example, is a symptom of increased metabolism and is not dangerous; its constructive nature promotes the free elimination of poisons through the skin.

Hildegard recognizes the greatest health-destroying factor is an excess of harmful body juices (*mali, noxi* and *infirmi humores*). They develop from overeating, nutritional poisons (see

Chapter Eight), raw diet, environmental poisons, a lack of good personal characteristics or virtues, and emotional poisons. Worry, troubles, rushing, stress, sadness, and anger increase black bile, a blood poison, which either leads to an outburst of anger or to a stifling reaction of suppression. The art of Hildegard medicine consists of either not allowing these body poisons to develop, or of conducting them expertly out of the body.

All Hildegard remedies are much more effective following a fasting therapy and bloodletting, according to Hildegard. Bloodletting is the universal healing method for all chronic disorders, as well as a prophylactic remedy for maintaining health. Every Hildgard friend is encouraged to have a yearly bloodletting, following Hildegard's precise procedures. Approximately one cup (150 milliliters) of blood is let during one of the six days starting with the full moon. The blood must run out by itself without suction until the black color changes to red. By this simple procedure, the sickness-causing black bile is removed and the body's own defense system activated.

Cupping is a method of conducting sicknesses out of the body through the skin. Wherever waste products or deposits settle in the body and cause inflammation and pain, cupping can be applied to eliminate these harmful substances. Cupping is primarily indicated for headaches, migraine, asthma, angina pectoris, and gall bladder or kidney stone attacks. It is especially effective against rheumatic pains, lumbago, sciatic pains, neuralgia, intervertebral and joint pains, varicose veins, and circulatory problems.

It is not surprising that Hildegard recommends the sauna as an effective remedy for the prevention and cure of arthritis, especially for corpulent patients. In the sweet chestnut sauna a person can sweat out his arthritis as well as a fit of anger or impatience.

A person who is plagued by arthritis and therefore furious, because arthritis is always connected with anger, should cook the leaves, shells, and nuts in water [to a sweet chestnut extract] and use it in the sauna. The person should do this often and the arthritis will leave, and the person will have mild and good senses again.   (PL 1226 C)

One needs at least ten sauna applications once or twice a

week. The sweet chestnut sauna is tried and proven for joint and muscular rheumatism, but it should never be used during an active attack or in cases of acute inflammation.

Arthritic patients, who are sensitive and inclined to neurosis, psychosis, or even schizophrenia, should take an oat sauna. The oat extract, poured on the hot stones, is inhaled and helps a person, above all, to find sleep naturally. The person's overstrained nerves have to recover during sleep. Patients showed marked improvement after ten sauna applications combined with the schizophrenia diet and nerve tea. (See Chapter Eleven.)

But whoever is arthritic and has a split mind from it and has crazy thoughts, so that the person goes mad from them, should pour the watery oat extract on the stones in the sauna. The person should do this often and will regain health again. (PL 1131 A)

In a similar way, thin people with weak supportive tissues are helped by a hot bath. Hildegard advises the addition of fresh spring fern for a wonderful, relaxing effect.

The fern contains much power, namely that the devil avoids it. It has certain energy which is like sun energy. . .Whoever suffers from gout should take fern when it is green and cook it in water (five to ten fern fronds in five quarts of water) and bathe often in this water bath, and the gout will leave. (PL 1148 B/C)

Barley baths are helpful for skinny, weak patients, when the muscles are shrinking or weakening because of a lack of exercise.

And whoever is so sick that the whole body is weak should cook barley in rapidly boiling water, pour the water in a tub, and bathe in it. This the person should do often, until cured and the [muscle] tissue grows stronger and healthy. (PL 1131 B)

Saunas and hot baths are very helpful, relaxing, and enjoyable, as long as they are not overdone. Especially during the winter, used in moderation once or twice a week, saunas and baths strengthen the whole body and activate the power of defense.

Compresses for various rheumatic pains can be just as reliable as a cortisone shot. Soft tissue rheumatism, lumbago, sciatic pain, or any other such as arthritis deformans will be helped with a compress of parsley and rue heated in olive oil.

A person with soft flesh and, because of excessive drinking, plagued by gout somewhere in the body, should take parsley and four times as

111

much rue and heat it in olive oil, or if the person has no olive oil, he or she can also take billy goat's fat. The herbs [after dripping] are placed hot on the painful places and tied with a bandage. (CC 213, 20)

The rue compress should be applied at least one-half hour and helps even in severe cases with pain and restriction of movement.

An ash-leaves compress is effective for severe arthritic pains in fingers, knees, hips and, if necessary, on the whole body.

If someone is plagued by rheumatism on the side, or on any of the limbs, as if all the limbs were broken and bruised, this person should cook ash leaves in water. After the patient is lying down on a linen cloth, wrap this person in the cooked, warm ash leaves, especially on the painful places. Do this often and he or she will feel better. (PL 1237 C)

Another compress recommended by Hildegard is the wheat compress, which is excellent for back pains, intervertebral pains, lumbago and sciatic pains. Depending on the size of the pain area, two to six pounds of wheat are boiled in two to six quarts of water for twenty minutes. Strain and put the hot wheat kernels on a folded towel in bed. Rest for two to three hours upon these hot kernels, being careful not to burn, once a day for five to ten days. As a reward after this treatment, drink a glass of galangal wine. This is prepared from one glass of wine and one teaspoon of powdered galangal, boiled, and eventually sweetened with honey. The wheat kernel compress is a great help where other treatments have failed, and should definitely be tried before a patient undergoes back surgery.

And whoever has pains in the back or loins should cook wheat kernels in water and lay them warm on the place that hurts and the warmth of the wheat will drive away the powers of that sickness. (PL 1129 C)

Through the Hildegard arthritis treatment, beginning with fasting, a person can be freed from physical and spiritual poisons and wastes. Fasting develops powerful healing and regenerating forces for protection and for defense. Hildegard calls this force "bravery."

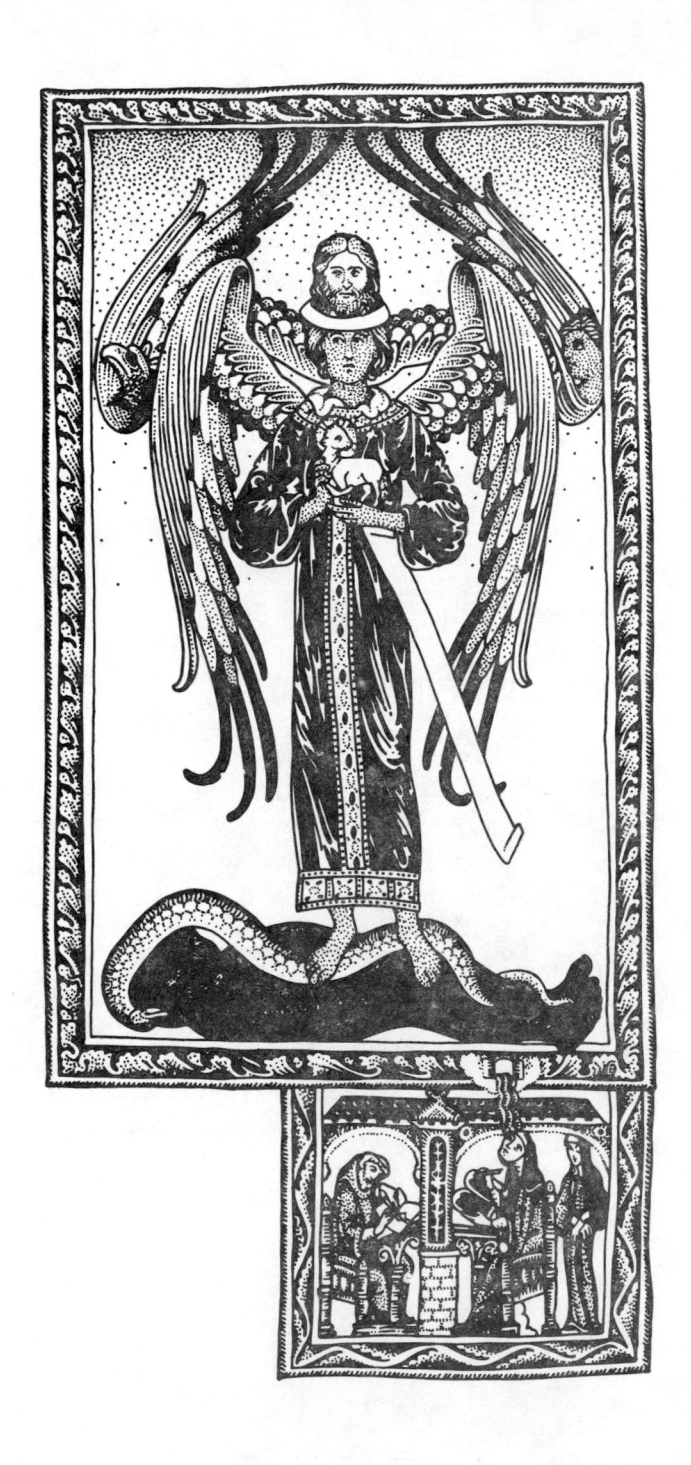

Chapter Fourteen

CANCER

LIFE GONE WILD

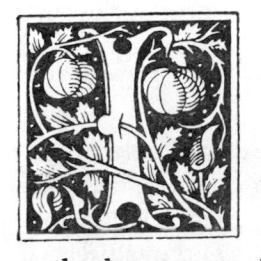

t is astonishing that Hildegard of Bingen described the cause, development, and treatment of cancer 800 years ago. She named the emotional reasons provoking this disease and how they make themselves felt in the molecular structure of the body itself. She even indicated remedies and methods to treat and prevent cancer, especially if one discovers it early enough during the time of the so-called precancer.

In the last fifty years, several Nobel prizes have been awarded and billions of dollars spent for cancer research. Modern science, nevertheless, cannot explain how cancer originates, how it grows (Cleveland State Law Review 1984/85) or how it can be healed. Medical science has no single remedy against cancer, nor will it have in the near future. The causes of cancer cannot be determined by today's medical science.

Depending on the type of tumor and the strength of immune resistance, nearly thirty years pass for a single tumor cell to grow into a tumor one centimeter in diameter, which already contains one billion tumor cells. Not until this late phase can the tumor be discovered through "early diagnosis." By then both patient and doctor can only react defensively with aggressive measures like operation, radiation, and chemotherapy— alternatives which are risky, unpleasant, and dangerous. In addition, these particular methods of treatment are associated with the greatest loss of quality of life. To this, a loss of appetite, sleeplessness, mutilation of the body, impotence, hopelessness, and despair must be added. No wonder that today over half the patients treated would rather die than go on living under such circumstances.

As long as the real reasons for the development of cancer are not taken into account, the number of cancer patients will increase. In 1900, cancer was the eighth leading cause of death, accounting for only four percent of deaths, with infectious diseases such as influenza, pneumonia, tuberculosis, and infectious gastrointestinal diseases far outranking it. Today, however, cancer accounts for about twenty percent of total U.S. mortality, second only to heart disease. The American Cancer Society estimated that 965,000 new cases of cancer would be diagnosed in 1987. The ACS also estimated 483,000 (more than 1300 per day) people would die from cancer in 1987.

Cancer is described by Hildegard as one of the 24 elementary original sicknesses (CC 54,21). Elementary original sicknesses are caused by the destruction of the four elements, which radically changes the whole order of human life and misdirects it. Some elementary disturbances are bad decisions regarding life style, dietary mistakes (kitchen poisons) or even environmental influences such as industrialization, pollution, or radioactive fallout.

The result of a disturbed juice and metabolic balance is a disturbed protein synthesis. Malignant cells produce large quantities of carcinogenic protein, so that the whole body swells and becomes poisoned. As the cancer cells grow, they replace healthy cells. Cancer cells devour substances important to life, like proteins and amino acids, so that the person wastes away and finally dies from anemia.

Hildegard's concept corresponds with the most modern scientific theories about cancer growth:

1. Uncontrolled growth.
2. Killing of host cells, either through local dissemination in the supportive tissues or,
3. Dissemination throughout the whole body to daughter cells (metastasis).

Preliminary symptoms are burping and hiccoughs.

Hildegard writes:

Whenever dryness or warmth, which make slime [livor] out of

116

moisture and foam, exceed their limit, then they produce loud burping and hiccoughs in people. In like manner, cancer can also develop in people and provoke viruses [vermes] to devour them. Moreover, they cause the body cells to swell into misshapen sores, so that through the growing tumor one arm or leg becomes larger than the other. When they do this for long, with no letup from the pestilence, the person cannot live long.

(CC 54, 21)

In the last 100 years, modern science has confirmed Hildegard's cancer concept step by step, without clearly recognizing it as such and utilizing its therapeutic possibilities.

In the nineteenth century, people saw a direct connection between chronic physical irritation (wounds, scars, ulcers) and the development of cancer cells. Although this cancer theory is no longer up-to-date, constant pressure and pain can cause tumors.

Later, people thought that small germs (parasites, bacteria, viruses) caused cancer. Hildegard writes about the very smallest worms and "lice" which can create cancer. Dr. Johannes Fibinger received a Nobel prize for this discovery in the 1920's. Interestingly, viral causes of cancer have been isolated in animals, but no virus has been seen in humans as yet.

Another cancer theory suggests that submicroscopic cancer cells are latent in every organism. At any time they can break loose through a tumor-creating occurrence, but they can also be kept under control by resistance of the body (immune system). Every person has his or her own sleeping cancer "pet," which can become a wild animal, if wakened through unfavorable circumstances. (J. Hackethal)

A kind of cancer-virus activation, its maturation (bursting open) and dispersal throughout the whole body as Hildegard describes it, has been confirmed by many researchers. Professor Günther Enderlain discovered a cancer microorganism in 1920, which he called "endobiotic." He described its development from the primary phase, through the bacterial phase, to the fungal phase in the final stage, which then infests the whole organism. According the Enderlein, cancer is not a conventional contagious disease, but rather every cell is already infested by the hard-to-detect endobiants in the primary phase, and it depends on the

117

body's resistance whether cancer forms or not.

In 1932, Dr. Wilhelm von Brehmer recognized the cancer-producing virus, *Siphonospora polymorpha*, in the blood of cancer patients. The cancer virus itself is an invisible stage of the *Siphonospora polymorpha* which can be seen as either a ball-shaped or tube-shaped form, or even as a foamy substance. It attacks the red blood corpuscles, grows in them, and finally destroys them.

In similar fashion, malaria plasmodia also attack the red blood corpuscles and feed on them to such an extent that the patient will die of secondary anemia. Hildegard describes how the "worms" gnaw at the mucous lining of the intestines like intestinal parasites, and subsist not only on the intestinal contents, but also on the blood like bloodsuckers. Through micro-hemorrhaging (for example, the bursting of an intestinal blood vessel or through taking aspirin) blood gets into the intestine and activates the pathogen. It becomes virulent and enters the blood as a cancer virus. We call this particular process "activation."

The newest cancer theory states that cancer-producing substances, or carcinogens, might require additional substances to initiate the process. Some substances may act as initiators, while others act as promoters.

Just as Hildegard writes, this process takes place in the cell nucleus where cell replication takes place. The nucleus controls all cell functions, the cell metabolism, and the differentiation into a certain type of cell, such as a nerve cell or liver cell. Each cell must contain and transmit to daughter cells the instructions governing the cells' own metabolism. These instructions are contained in molecules of deoxyribose nucleic acid (DNA), which is found almost exclusively in the cell nucleus. DNA, in the form of a double helix with its control mechanism, was discovered by two other Nobel prize winners—James Dewey Watson and Francis Harry Crick—in 1962.

The DNA-double helix, resembling a spiral staircase, replicates itself by "unzipping" completely during the process of cell division, so that each daughter cell is a complete copy of all the information in the parent cell. DNA may also partially "unzip," and transcribe certain information to single stranded molecules

118

of ribonucleic acid (RNA). The strands of DNA are collected in chromosomes. Choromosomes functionally are divided into genes, the hereditary determinants of the genetic code.

Although scientists do not exactly know what causes cancer in humans, they do know that cancer is a multiple-step process. The disease seems to develop progressively through a number of stages, each of which can be influenced by chemicals, environmental factors interacting with host factors such as nutrition, hormone levels, etc.

Another important requirement for the development of cancer is an excess of black bile, the so-called "melanche," which increases under stress, agitation, worries, fear, frustration, or sorrow. This black bile joins forces with other "bad juices," creating a very bad septic slime or ferment.

As we know today from the famous Nobel prize winner, Otto Warburg, and his cancer experiment, the respiration of cancer cells is damaged. A decreased oxygen supply suffices, so that the cells switch from breathing oxygen (aerob) to a ferment exchange (anaerob). Cancer cells need no oxygen and secure their energy from fermentation, whereby lactic acid, as well as decaying and poisonous substances, are produced and the surroundings overacidify. Lactic acid also develops by sudden overexertion of the muscles, and causes the sore muscles familiar to everyone.

Hildegard lists the stomach, intestines, and supportive tissues (between skin and flesh) as the kitchen producing this fermentation and poison. These substances lie as capsulated buds (rheumatoid centers), or sleeping dogs, in the supportive tissues. From time to time, during an unfavorable state with a lack of resistance, the patient suffers pain attacks coming from these centers. "They torture the person with great severity, as if they were biting and gnawing," describes Hildegard vividly. These distribution centers are not filled with germs, but rather with so-called "crystalline viruses," which still have no life of their own. This statement from Hildegard has been verified by modern science.

Wendell M. Stanley received a Nobel prize in 1946 for the discovery of highly infectious viruses, or pathogenic agents, which exist as crystals on the border between active and inactive nature and can be isolated. These tumor-causing viruses, or oncogenes, require a host for their growth and reproduction.

Hildegard even describes the secret of the development of tumor-causing viruses in cancer, which we call activated cancer. A foam comes into being and spreads throughout the whole body (dispersion centers, metastasis, daughter cells) causing the person pain.

During cell reproduction, poison and fermenting substances (protein toxins) may be built into the DNA-double helix as the wrong building material. Through this mistake, not normal cells, but cancer cells with their own metabolism are produced.

Now dangerous cancer viruses bubble out of the DNA in the cell nucleus, which Hildegard calls especially vicious, tiny organisms, *perdiculi* (literally, "lice"). How else should Hildegard have called these small destroyers 800 years ago, when pathogenic agents have only been identified under the microscope and called bacteria and viruses within the last century?

Cancer viruses are similar to aggressive pirates, who capture a ship and then force the crew to work for them. The body has been forced to produce only cancer cells through the virus-protein synthesis. Now they overrun the whole body and flood it with alien protein poisons.

Hildegard's description of the complete cancer mechanism, which modern medicine has only begun to solve, is presented in her simple, vivid language:

Persons with an average physique, neither too fat nor too thin, usually have a well-balanced household of body juices and are seldom struck by vicht [precancer], because the juices causing this affliction are not excessively present. But those who are too fat or too thin possess excessive bad juices [mali humores], because they do not have the right structure and balance in themselves. These bad juices rise occasionally from the heart, liver, lungs, stomach, and intestines, and get to the black bile and create smoke [fumi] there and a very bad slime [pessimum livor], somewhat like standing water that floods and overflows the shore with rotten silt. This slime reaches either the stomach or the intestines, or some other place between skin and flesh, sticks there and tortures the person with great severity, as if it were biting and gnawing. It does not yet have the vitality to force its way into the person, but only a kind of caustic acid. It looks like buds which lie in the cells of the person like lentils in the tissues. Sometimes it stretches itself in length, another time it rolls itself together like a ball, similar to an egg yolk, and sometimes it produces a kind of foam which spreads throughout the whole body and causes pain. But whenever this foam penetrates into the stomach, a kind of worms bubble out of it [virulent activated cancer], from which especially vicious tiny organisms develop in the cells. . . (CC 157, 19)

As Hildegard describes, activated cancer, from non-reproducing cancer-causing substances to virulent tumor-causing viruses, takes place in the stomach and intestinal tract by way of hemorrhages. After that, the cancer viruses force their way into the whole body and can create tumors. In this final stage the cancer growth is extremely difficult to treat, if at all, and then only with very aggressive methods such as surgery, radiation, and chemotherapy.

RECOGNIZING PRECANCER

Healing cancer begins with early recognition in the precancer phase; this is the key to prevention! The symptoms of precancer are easy to recognize, once they are known. The person complains about a lack of appetite and insomnia, tiredness, weakness, and a loss of vitality. Especially characteristic are the constantly returning rheumatic ailments such as lumbago, sciatic pains, stiff neck, as well as heart pains, cramps, and colics. Blood sedimentation is greatly increased.

Years before the outbreak of cancer can be detected, one can observe under the microscope remarkable phenomena in urine sediment. In phase contrast, or after coloring with orceine, numerous granulate and killer cells are perceptible. They can be identified as special leukocytes and take on a characteristic form as the disease progresses.

In the first stage of precancer, one can see isolated killer cells which are bigger than normal leukocytes and possess a closed, well-defined form like a mulberry. (Robert Heintz et al., *Harnsediment Atlas*, Ill. 16, Thieme Verlag.) On the inside, one recognizes clearly a dark crescent-formed center. The cells move characteristically according to the Brown molecular movement.

In the second stage, one can observe numerous cells in whose closed form globular cavities are found. They have been labeled pregnant leukocytes.

In the third stage, the cell wall is not longer closed but ruptured; we call these cells "exploded leukocytes." Small round bubbles hang on the cell like suction cups on the tentacles of an octopus. This stage of activated cancer can be observed in patients with an advanced condition of illness.

THE TREATMENT OF PRECANCER

Because precancer is a general illness affecting the whole body, a sensible treatment must also involve the whole person. Several specific possibilites of treatment come from Hildegard and help the patient to prevent cancer, or, at least, to bring it to a standstill.

The treatment of precancer begins with the treatment of all chronic localities of inflammation and infection, such as teeth, tonsils, sinuses, gall bladder, kidney, and bladder. Besides remedies for specific organs out of the great Hildegard therapy, a correctly performed bloodletting helps in every case. It improves basic metabolism and stimulates the body's own healing capacity, which has been blocked by black bile and bad, sickness-making juices.

Bloodletting has the following characteristics: anti-inflamatory, spasmolytic (stopping cramps), antidyskrastic (improving basal metabolism) and bloodcleansing (removing black bile). Especially in cases of severe chronic illnesses, bloodletting has brought about cures where today's modern school of medicine has had no success.

By observing the phenomena of the blood which has been let, a sophisticated analysis is possible. Cloudiness, color, and quality of the blood plasma and serum give indications about the further course of the illness. Specific indications can be observed concerning signs of inflammation, state of mood according to the quantity of black bile, and state of nutrition according to the quantity of blood fat and waxy overlap of the blood plasma.

After bloodletting, the duckweed elixir therapy is begun, since, following detoxification, it can have its full effect. Duckweed elixir is very difficult to prepare and if it is to be made properly, requires a great gallenic skill. The honeywine extract is made out of cinnamon, sage, ginger, fennel, rue, white pepper, tormentil, field mustard *(Sinapis arvensis)*, burdock *(Arctium lappa)*, and wild bedstraw *(Galium aparine)*, and is filtered hot into the duckweed *(Lemna minor)*. One sherry glass full (twenty milliliters) is taken before breakfast and again before bedtime for three months.

Hildegard describes the effect of duckweed elixir in her own language with an exact and understandable explanation:

Precancer develops from warm and cold bad juices, but more from the cold than from the warm ones. . .The combination of various herbs in the right proportion lessens the false warm and false cold juices, which cause colic. If the person takes duckweed elixir before eating and at bedtime, this will prevent bad juices from developing on an empty stomach, or from foods after eating. (CC 209, 22 ff)

Some of Hildegard's knowledge can be proved by scientific methods. Herbs such as ginger, tormentil *(Potentilla tormentilla)*, and bedstraw stimulate the body's own powers of resistance. The immune system protects us from external poisons like bacteria, viruses, toxins, and allergens, as well as from pathogens in the body itself, which cause sicknesses. Because the immune system is effective in all fields, it registers every change in its environment without differentiating between inside and outside.

With the support of the immune system, we protect our microcosmos inside the body and activate ourselves and our health towards the macrocosmos on the outside. Our strongest weapon in the fight against severe epidemics like cancer, AIDS, or whatever technological civilization and the destruction of creation may bring about in the future, is our body's own immune system. Hildegard calls this weapon God's military *(militia dei)*.

Stimulants which effect our immune system are the energies from the four elements, fire, air, water and earth, as found in climate, movement and exercise, breathing, baths or showers, and sunshine. Energies from earth come from herbal medicines and correct nutrition by way of the Hildegard diet with its most important component: the age-old grain, spelt.

Spelt intensifies the power of resistance, beginning in the

intestinal tract, and gives the whole body nourishment of high quality. Spelt also removes dangerous poisonous substances and deposits, and improves the complete general health of the person. During precancer, a patient should do without animal protein, replacing it with spelt two to three times a day, although Hildegard does recommend deer liver, especially for persons with precancer.

Most important for effective treatment in the fight against cancer viruses is the removal of their supportive terrain, or culture medium. This principle has always belonged to the most successful methods of treatment by natural remedies which are in total opposition to those of school medicine. School medicine gets rid of external pathogens by conducting an attack with antibiotics, without considering the body's own defenses. Today, utter helplessness is evident in the face of the cancer problem and AIDS; natural-science-oriented medicine has landed in a blind alley.

The newest medical research proves that stimulation of the body's immune system is ultimately the only way to protect people from new plagues. Hildegard medicine acquires scientific accuracy—not required for treatment, but necessary for medical science—through the results of this research. These studies, publicized recently at a special congress for methods of natural remedies, enable even medical doctors to use these successful methods in their practices.

Not only Hildegard, but also modern scientific epidemiological studies, recognize many inner and outer factors which help promote cancer. Hildegard names 35 psychological risk factors as handicaps producing sickness-causing reactions. In accordance with Hildegard's psychotherapeutic book, *Book of Life's Merits*, and the psychological studies of the Cancer Research Institute in Heidelberg, West Germany, it is extremely risky and dangerous to live a life filled with sorrow, worry, fear, chronic stress, and hurry—as in the daily rush. Especially cancer-provoking are chronic hopelessness or desperation, doubt, unbelief, world-weariness, and the pessimistic sadness of the world.

The Heidelberg psychologists even found that the calloused

person, whose faith has dried up, is the one to be afflicted most frequently by cancer. The militant atheists, who live at the greatest distance from God, together with the tolerant atheists, follow. The persons with the least cancer were those with a "spontaneous religiousness," who live from the strength and joy of their faith.

IS THERE A
TYPICAL CANCER PERSONALITY?

Besides psychological risk factors, social factors also play a role in provoking cancer, which have their primary source in the character of the person. We already know that almost everyone has cancer cells in the body, which are kept under control by the body's own powers of resistance. Modern cancer research has found out how much these powers of resistance are influenced by individual characteristics.

The typical cancer personality is characterized by cancer researchers as follows: Most cancer patients are lovable persons, cooperative and helpful, flexible and self-sacrificing. They acknowledge religion and authority and are prepared to take their place in society and carry responsibility. Nevertheless, they are not able to master the crises in their lives, so that through the loss of mate or goal they collapse with laming fatigue, doubt, and chronic hopelessness. Their life is marked by frustration, inner emptiness, and aimlessness.

In order to forecast cancer, one must take not only the loss and depression theory into account, but also childhood experiences. Disturbances experienced at home in early childhood are sometimes repressed as unresolved conflicts in the subconscious. Some such disturbances are a lack of nest warmth from father and mother, loss of a parent, or a divorce. Whenever these unresolved conflicts are repeated at a grown-up age through the loss of a mate or one's own divorce, old wounds break open again which had never healed under the surface. This can lead to serious crises of life, to depressions and hopelessness. If these crises are not resolved, but rather swallowed in silent grief, the powers of resistance may weaken and cancer may break out.

Hildegard's psychotherapy, with its pairs of virtues and

vices, points us in a new direction. Desperation asks, "Who could comfort me? What do I have left, other than death? I have no more joy in good, because there is nothing good on the Earth!" And Hope answers, "If you look for good outside of God, no one can help you anymore!"

The newest cancer research can even prove that there is a direct relationship between spiritual protective factors like hope, joy, and affection, which strengthens the defensive powers of the immune system. Hildegard speaks about the *militia dei*, God's military or spiritual powers of resistance, which can cause hormonal fluctuations and thereby mobilize healing powers

Numerous scientific examinations have also shown that severe psychic stress, like hopelessness, fear, and doubt, stimulates the hormone production in the central nervous system. Through a high hormone level in the blood (cortisone, insulin, histamine) the body's resistance can be so weakened that the development of cancer is provoked.

THE BEST CANCER TREATMENT

According to Hildegard, the key to successful cancer therapy is early detection and treatment beginning in the precancer state. Modern preventative examinations only recognize last stage cancer, when two-thirds of the malignant process is completed. Although an operable tumor should be carefully removed by surgery on principle, if one does not want to be accused of malpractice, every surgical incision into a cancer growth brings the danger of metastasis development. Most metastases begin to grow during the first operation, when the cancer viruses have become virulent. Four out of five patients die from metastases and not from the first tumor. The unguarded, tissue-sample excision, or cancer operation, is therefore also malpractice.

We recommend all patients who must undergo a cancer operation only to go ahead under protection of yarrow (sneezewort, *Achillea millifolium*). Three days before the operation they should take three pinches of yarrow powder daily, first in fennel tea, and later in warm wine or heart wine. After the operation, they should continue with the same amount for eight more days. Through yarrow protection, metastases almost never develop, and the wound will heal smooth and quickly without infection. Yarrow treatment also protects against radiation damage to healthy tissues. This is Hildegard's best protection against wound infection; yarrow can also be used externally.

In her *Physica*, Hildegard writes:

Whoever is wounded in the inside of the body, whether it came through a knife or an inner injury, should powder yarrow and drink it in warm water. When better, the person should keep on drinking the powder in warm wine until healed. (PL 1175 D)

Cancer is not a localized sickness, which one can simply cut out with a knife. Rather it is a serious general inner sickness which seizes the entire organism. For this reason, orthodox medicine recommends cytostatica (chemotherapy) and radiation after a radical cancer operation, through which severe side-effects arise, as well as damage, which may lead to invalidism and the loss of quality of life.

The healing goal of orthodox medicine is survival from this procedure for up to five years. Many patients suffer so much from the aftereffects of treatment that they would rather die than continue living. This is without regarding the fact that within a short time tumors may develop again in many patients.

Hildegard's cancer remedy, anguillan, is made from a complicated honeywine-vinegar extract out of eel gall, ginger, long pepper, basil (*Ocimum basilicum*), ivory powder, and the powder from vulture beak. The acquisition and production of this drug involves enormous difficulties. We had to wait five years for the chance to obtain a vulture, which had been killed in an accident, from a Hildegard friend. Vultures are protected worldwide as an endangered species, and may not be hunted.

The use of the vulture as a medicine can be traced back four-thousand years. In the twelfth and thirteenth centuries, vulture beak was already described as a remedy in the first German medical book. The attractiveness of the vulture drug, and the relevance of its prescription and therapy, caused the wide circulation of medieval vulture treatises (Joachim Stümer, Von deme Gire, *Untersuchungen zu Einer Altdeutschen Drogenmonographie des Hochmittelalters*, Würzburger Medizinische Forschung, Bd. 12, 1978).

127

Hildegard recommends this cancer remedy for persons who have been internally damaged by cancer viruses:

The viruses in the body will get sick and die and the infested fatty tissue will regenerate. The warmth and bitter acid of the eel gall weaken the viruses; the warmth of vinegar acid dissolves them; the warmth and dryness of ivory causes them to dry up; the vulture beak kills them, because it is cold and poisoned through many kinds of carcasses; besides, it is soaked from the sweat of the brain [sudore]. (CC 210, 30)

Everywhere where cystostatica are being used, a holistic therapy with Hildegard's cancer remedy, anguillan, can also be taken into consideration. Anguillan has no harmful side effects. For a course of treatment, it is used homeopathically raised to a higher power as D_6, D_{12} and D_{30}. It is recommended to take ten drops six times a day in heart wine before and after eating, beginning with D_6, later D_{12} and finally D_{30}. The treatment should be continued four to six weeks accompanied by the Hildegard spelt diet. For optimal results, the diet should omit the four kitchen poisons (strawberries, peaches, plums, and leeks), animal protein, and nightshade plants like potatoes, tomatoes, and green peppers.

FROM THE TUMOR—BREAST CANCER

Hildegard devotes a separate chapter to the development and treatment of breast cancer, in which context she uses the word "tumor" or "growth". The start of breast cancer is described as being caused by "worms", which links it to other causes of cancer. An excess of good and bad juices (*boni et mali humores*) can trigger growth and lead to swellings in the breast.

Through various [good and bad] juices the tissues and vessels of a person will swell, just as flour is stimulated and rises through yeast. The juices which come from heart, liver, lungs, stomach, and other inner organs may become sluggish, greasy, and only lukewarm, if they are mixed together incorrectly and have developed excessively. If they remain in the person, they will cause sickness; whereas if they escape, they will make the person healthy. (CC 154, 18)

For harmless cysts in the connective tissues (a form of precancer) Hildegard recommends violet salve, which in many cases makes these lumps disappear. Hildegard even allows the tumors to ripen. We recommend, as a matter of principle and from fear of malpractice, to allow the tumor to be surgically removed under protection of yarrow. The operation should be performed as carefully as possible with preservation of the breast and lymph glands. Postoperative treatment to prevent recurrance includes duckweed elixir and violet salve.

Whenever such juices attack a person on any particular place, so that one or more sores [ulcus] are formed, then the person should let them ripen, so that they can discharge. Then they will not cause still greater pains, as if they had remained on the inside. As soon as the juices have drained in the ripened stage, then the person should go ahead with a violet salve treatment.

Take violets, press out their juice, and strain it through a cloth. Add olive oil one-third the weight of the juice and take just as much billy goat's fat as violet juice. Boil everything in a clean pot and prepare a salve.

Salve the body parts all around, and also right there where the cancer and other viruses [vermes] are devouring the person. The viruses will die when they have tasted the salve. One should rub it into other sores [ulcera] too, which hurt the person. If anyone is plagued by headaches, this person should rub it right over the forehead.(CC 204, 25)

The scientific recognition of Hildegard medicine is not necessary for its effectiveness. The believing Hildegard friend knows that this medicine comes from God's wisdom and is on the highest level of perception, which needs no human justification. Nevertheless, already over 100 herbal drugs have been acknowledged as effective and harmless by the German Food and Drug Administration (Bundesgesundheitsamt). This is based on monographs on such substances as galangal, rue, agrimonia, etc., which have been written with our cooperation.

The demand for exact scientific proof of effectiveness is unfortunately, for many people today, absolutely necessary, because science has become a pseudoreligion. In spite of the fact that much of the exact scientific knowledge of today will become the errors of tomorrow, the label "scientifically proven" has become the sales argument of the pharmaceutical industry, and also of many doctors. The so-called objective clinical proof through specific clinical studies is regrettably not only a question of "pure science," but also of money and power, these proofs being proclaimed by the so-called "opinion leaders."

For this reason, many of the Hildegard remedies are not yet scientifically recognized, with the tragic result that health insurance only pays for their achievements in certain cases. It is the responsibility of the many patients who have been helped through Hildegard medicine to influence politicians, so that the cost of these natural remedies may be reimbursed by insurance companies for the good of public welfare.

Through her description of the development and treatment of sicknesses, Hildegard presents new theories, hitherto unknown to the world at large. In an almost ideal way, she fulfills the ideal claim: no sickness without a remedy. Hereby many cancer patients are finally able to free their powers of self-healing, which otherwise would have remained hidden and unused, through new courage and hope.

After the many errors and confusion of cancer research, Hildegard gives us a clear concept for cancer prevention and early recognition during the long preliminary stage of precancer. During this time, the cancer viruses can usually be destroyed, or at least brought to a standstill.

Chapter Fifteen

FASTING

CREATING YOUR OWN SPIRITUALITY

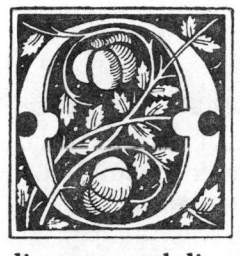 ver the last few centuries, humanity has become more and more materialistic. Most people fight for their own survival, and forget the millions of others who starve. Exploitation of the Earth has polluted the atmosphere and contaminated the soil. All of earthly creation is suffering from wars, diseases, and disasters.

Hildegard writes in her *Scivias*, part III, vision 5:

The rest of creation cries out and complains loudly against such inhumanity, because the more vile human nature is, in its short existence, the more it is a rebel against God.

Again in her book, *Liber Vitae Meritorum*, part III, she says how the four elements are crying out to God, as nature pleads:

We cannot run anymore and cannot fulfill our destiny, because humanity is defiling us with sinful deeds and turning us around. All the winds are mortified and the air spews out filth that people dare not breathe. But God will clean the elements with the Divine broom and punish humanity until it looks toward its heavenly parent once more.

Hildegard foresees in her *Scivias* a new age of spirituality in which Christians will finally live in their promised land. She symbolically describes five beasts:

1. The Fiery Dog:
represents the injustice of Christianity, the separation of the Eastern and Western churches, including the reformation and the discovery of America.

131

2. The Red Lion:
stands for the blood shed during the religious wars and
strife among Christians, including the world wars.

3. The Pale Horse:
represents the time of change from the love of luxury
and materialism towards spirituality; within this time,
Christians will find peace on Earth and goodwill among
humans.

4. The Black Pig:
represents a time of crisis during which the Christian
faith dries up.

5. The Grizzly Wolf:
represents the period of the anti-Christ.

When all this has come to pass, then Christ shall return for the
Last Judgment.

In order to prepare for the future, we must set up new pri-
orities, based on new values to overcome materialism. (Luke
12:30 NEV) "...You are not to set your mind on food and drink;
you are not to worry. For all these are things for the heathen to
run after; but you have a father who knows that you need them.
No, set your mind upon his kingdom and all the rest will come
to you as well."

More than the toxins in the food we eat, the impurities in the
heart must disappear. (Mark 7:18) "...Nothing that goes from
outside into a person can defile, because it does not enter into the
heart but into the stomach, and so passes out into the drain."
Thus Jesus declared all foods clean.

He went on, "It is what comes out of a person that defiles.
For from inside, out of the heart, come evil thoughts, acts of for-
nication, of theft, murder, adultery, ruthless greed, and malice;
fraud, indecency, envy, slander, arrogance, and folly; these evil
things all come from inside, and they defile the person."

In Hildegard's book of psychotherapy, she describes 35 vices
and virtues of thought-patterns, as layers in the subconscious.
One can analyze oneself and discover one's own spiritual personality pattern. For 29 vices, the dark sides of people, Hildegard
suggests fasting as a universal remedy in order to achieve spirituality. Since food represents the materialistic part of us, fasting
permits these blockages to surface and release, so that one

attunes to the soul.

Hildegard warns not to fast by the following vices:

(1) love of the world
(13) melancholy (depression)
(14) immoderation
(16) arrogance
(26) uncertainty (inconsistency)
(35) grief of the world

In order to prepare for the new millenium and to be a spiritual individual, we must release the burden of our vices, influence of our enemies, and move toward the new world of hope, love, and harmony. No human being can contain all 35 virtues, so it is important to concentrate on one virtue, like peace. We need lots of peace angels today. The peace angel has two wings that represent high days and low days, when peace is more difficult to maintain. Peace says to Contention:

I am a remedy [medicine] for all the conditions you have caused. I heal where you destroy. I declare all these things, such as wars, as unjustified, self-defeating, and an everlasting contention. I am a mountain [overseeing all conflicts so that I can promptly intervene]. I am full of fragrance like myrrh and incense. [Peace creates an aura of tranquility.] (LVM II)

During a fast, everyone will receive two strong healing forces. The first is unlimited energy for holistic health, strong creative forces (*operarii Dei*), and a build-up of spiritual potential. The second is the power of defense (*fortisima militia*, the divine military) to fortify the psychosomatic resistance necessary to overcome degenerative diseases, such as cancer, AIDS, and multiple sclerosis.

A beneficial side effect of fasting is the release of poison and waste products both in the tissues and throughout the body. Fasting effectively stimulates the building and growth of new cells, restoring health and rejuvenating the body. After the first three days, the body will nurture itself. When nutrition is required, it will burn and digest from its own inner storehouse. First attended are those cells and tissues which are dead, diseased, or damaged, such as tumorous cells, arterial sclerotic plaques, and rubbish in body and mind. This accelerates the force of regeneration. The level of blood cholesterol and blood pressure will return to normal.

During fasting, a vast amount of toxins and wastes (uric acids) leave the body and in so doing retoxify the blood for a very short time. Sometimes fasters experience a fasting crisis; retoxification may cause headache, pain, dizziness, or weakness.

To begin, group fasting is recommended under the supervision of an expert for no longer than one week to ten days at a time. Therapeutic fasting for longer periods must be done in a clinic. It is best to start with two to three days of preparation, eating only cooked spelt, vegetables, fresh fruit, and garden lettuce. Tobacco, coffee, and alcohol, as well as unnecessary drugs are completely withdrawn. Consult your doctor for advice. It is the best way to quit smoking and drinking.

Fasting begins with an effective colon cleansing. The most common method has been with the help of a purgative such as Glauber's salt (1 ½ ounces Glauber's salt in one pint of water). Since Glauber's salt tastes awful, quickly drink a cup of herb tea and suck some slices of lemon. Five to ten hours later you will have several repeated bowel movements.

Instead of this harsh method, Hildegard suggests a purgative cookie made from a mixture of spices—ginger, zittwer (*Radix zedoariae*), and sweet wood licorice. Before eating this cookie, warm yourself in front of a fire if it is cold outside, and afterwards rest on your bed while remaining awake. Thereafter, walk slowly and do not let the cold overwhelm you. In this way the spices retain the good fluids, whereas the noxious ones (*noxi humores*) will leave the body.

You can also begin your fast without the purgative by administering a double enema. Take one pint of camomile tea water, hold it in, and release in five minutes. Repeat the same procedure with two pints and continue doing this daily before you go to bed. Enemas are essential during fasting, since toxic wastes would otherwise remain in the body and would be reabsorbed into the blood.

Weaknesses, or passing ailments, during the time of fasting can all be effectively treated with Hildegard remedies. Heart wine, taken as needed during fasting, has been discovered to permanently normalize not only high, but also low blood pressure. A second surprising discovery was the emergency drug, galangal, which immediately lowers high blood pressure, improves impaired circulation and prevents heart attacks. A bowl of "happy-making" fennel seeds provides the fasters with good breath and a clear vision.

Hildegard fasting is based on a total abstention from eating—just drinking plenty of herb teas, spelt coffee, fruit and vegetable juices, and lots of spring or well water, minimum of three quarts a day. Once a day, you should have a fasting soup. Take one cup of spelt per person, add three cups water, chopped carrots, beans, tomatoes, red beets, celery, and herbs. Boil for twenty to thirty minutes. Drain and only drink the liquid. This soup contains all the vital vitamins and minerals.

Your body will need plenty of exercise and *viriditas* from all four elements—fresh air, water, sunshine, and earth enjoyed through walks, or even mountain climbing. You may be surprised that after three days you feel strong and vital, with clarity of thought and even creativity. Fasting requires its own rules. Retreat from your daily routine—no telephone, peaceful surroundings, and people with supportive interest. The following plan was found helpful:

7:00 am:
wake up with dry brush massage; hot and cold showers.
7:30 am:
exercise; gymnastics.
8:00 am:
morning herb tea or spelt coffee.
12:00 noon:
hot fasting soup.
12:30 pm:
rest with a warm liver compress (a hot water bottle or towel on the liver area).
2:30 pm:
herb tea.
3:00 pm:
extended walk or hiking.
6:00 pm
fresh fruit or vegetable juice.

8:00 pm:
meditation, singing, playing, reading.
10:00 pm:
enema, warm shower, and rest.

HOW TO BREAK FAST
First Recovery Day

Breakfast:
spelt rice—add ½ cup spelt (may be coarsely ground) to
1 cup of water; boil for 20 to 30 minutes; spice with cinnamon, galangal, pellitory (*Anacyclus pyrethrum*) and
honey.
Eat and chew slowly; never overeat.
Noon Meal:
vegetable soup and a bowl of fresh chopped garden lettuce with 3 spoons spelt rice; a dressing of sunflower oil,
wine vinegar, and some brown sugar, without salt.
(See recipe in Chapter Eight).
Supper:
spelt bread—1 pound of spelt flour (whole grain wheat
flour); 3 teaspoons of spice (quendal—*Herba serpylli*,
galangal and pellitory); ½ package of yeast; 1 pint warm
water.
Knead the dough; leave the dough to rise for 1½ hours,
then bake in a hot oven for one hour. The bread spread
can be made out of cottage cheese with herbs or fresh
cheese, spiced with cumin.

Repeat this for one week in order to regain a perfectly normal digestion without the aid of laxatives. In order to continue
benefits for the future, maintain the Hildegard diet and exercise
positive spiritual values. It is a great way to prevent diseases and
degeneration of the body. It improves nerves and mental functioning, normalizes body and brain chemistry, and lowers blood
cholesterol and toxins.

At the end of the fast, one feels like a new person. Hildegard
writes:

*In humans, God has completed all divine work. . . not only the four
elements, fire, water, earth, and air are included in humans, but also the
virtues of the happy person.*

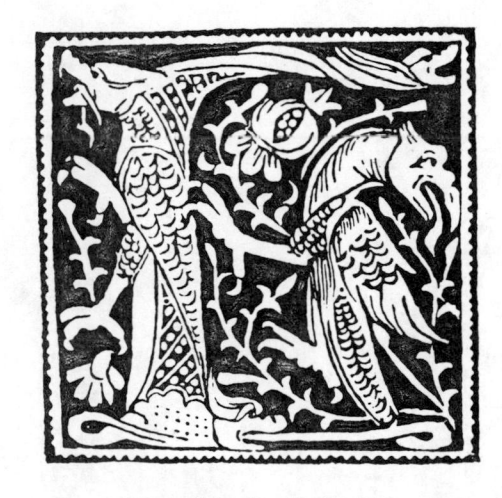

SAINT
HILDEGARD

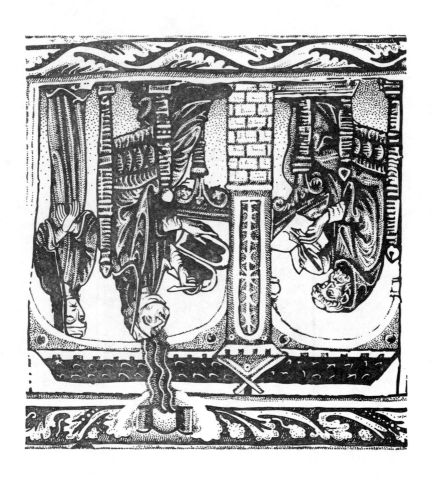

SAINT HILDEGARD
& HER MEDICINE

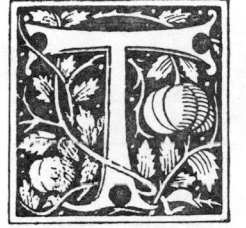his book marks the debut of Hildegard medicine in America. Hildegard medicine was completely forgotten for 800 years. Her medical books were never taken seriously, not even when her textbook of medicine, *Causae et Curae* (CC), was discovered 100 years ago in the Royal Library of Copenhagen, nor when her book of remedies, *Physica*, was translated into Latin by Cardinal Pitra.

Nobody would know that Hildegard medicine exists, if it had not been for the physician, Dr. Gottfried Hertzka. He practiced Hildegard medicine in Germany, rediscovered her medical knowledge and advice, and made them available for our age.

There are now many scholars studying Hildegard all over the world; but without medicine, Hildegard's work is only a torso with theological, mystical, or prophetical parts. For a total view of Hildegard, it is necessary to include her medicine.

St. Hildegard of Bingen was a great woman of the Middle Ages, a bright star in the firmament of western intellectual and spiritual history. The bright splendor that radiated throughout her whole life came from a mysterious phenomenon: the audio-vision transmitted to her imagination by divine command which carried the message of prophecy. That was her charisma, a fundamental quality of her life.

Hildegard was the most remarkable of mystics, for she never experienced ecstasies, or similar states of unconsciousness.

139

When Wilbert of Gembloux asked Hildegard for a detailed description of her charisma, the seventy-seven-year-old seer from the Rhine gave the monk the following information:

I see these things not with my external eyes, nor do I hear them with my external ears. I see them rather only in my soul with my bodily eyes wide open, so that I am never overcome by ecstatic unconsciousness, but see these things when I am awake during the day and during the night. The light that I see is not confined to space. It is much lighter than a cloud which bears the sun within it. I can recognize neither height nor length nor breadth in it. I am told it is the shadow of the living light [umbra lucis viventis]. In this light I sometimes, but not often, see another light which I am told is the living light [lux vivens]. When and how long I can see it I cannot say. But as long as I see it, all sadness and all fear are taken from me, so that I feel like a simple young girl and not like an old woman. (Pitra, see page xxvi)

Hildegard was born in 1098 at a country estate in Bermersheim near Alzey in Rheinhessen. Even as a child Hildegard possessed this unusual capability and saw things which other people could not see; for example, the coloring of a calf while still unborn, or pictures from far-away regions and out of the past. The tenth child of her noble parents, she was dedicated to God as their tithe from the time she was very young. Because of her wonderful gift and natural piousness, Hildegard's parents entrusted their eight-year-old daughter to the Benedictine sister, Jutta von Sponheim, at the Disibodenberg cloister near Kreuznach. The recluse, Jutta, taught her reading and writing, psalm singing, needlework, and music.

When Hildegard was sixteen, she became a nun at the Benedictine convent. After Jutta's death in 1136, Hildegard was unanimously chosen as the abbess, and she led the blossoming convent until her death in 1181.

Her life can be divided into two halves of approximately 35 years each. For the first 35 years she lived silently in the isolation of the daily life of the monastery. The second 35 years can be divided into five periods.

The first of these five periods began in 1141 when Hildegard was flooded and inflamed with an intense light from above, receiving her commission as a prophet. At all times of the day

140

and night she saw a heavenly screen in front of her, like a shimmering cloud of light containing words and pictures. She heard wonders and explanations coming from it and a heavenly voice told her to write down all she experienced.

Obedient and dedicated, Hildegard began to write her first theological work, *Scivias* (know the ways), which was a gift to her cloister, Disibodenberg. *Scivias*, published today in English, is the most complete documentation of Christian faith in which the secrets of God are described in words, images, and music. The prophecies found in *Scivias* were tested and verified by a papal committee supervised by St. Bernard Clairveaux. Pope Eugene III personally authorized and read from *Scivias* at the Trier synod in 1147. Overnight, Hildegard became famous.

In the second period from 1151 to 1159, an independent Hildegard founded her own convent on the Rupertsberg near Bingen. This convent attracted an increasing number of sisters, whom Hildegard trained in the Benedictine way of life. Rupertsberg became the meeting place of Europe! As if attracted by a magnet, thousands came to seek council from Hildegard.

At the same time, she started an extraordinary work comprised of seven books. *Liber Simplicus Medicinae*, (also called *Physica*), a handbook on nature, and *Liber Compositae Medicinae* (also called *Causae et Curae*), a handbook on medicine, were the first books. There followed a song book with 77 chants, hymns, antiphons, sequences, and responsories in a cycle entitled *Symphonia Harmonia Coelestium Revolutionum* (the harmonic symphony of cosmic revolutions).

In her concern for the kingdom of God, this great woman wrote 300 letters to people seeking advice. She corresponded with bishops, cardinals, abbots, emperors, popes, kings, clergymen, and people from various levels of society, both in Germany and abroad.

During this time she also wrote a book, *Lingua Ignota*, (the unknown language) which has not yet been decoded. This language contains 900 words and an alphabet of 23 letters, perhaps related in some way to the genetic code. In addition to these five works, she wrote a sixth book on the gospels, and a seventh, *Aphorisma*, her personal notebook.

141

From 1158 to 1163, the third period, Hildegard wrote her second theological book, *Liber Vitae Meritorum* (the book of life's merits), which could be called a handbook of life. This psychotherapeutical book describes the 35 layers of our subconscious, and 35 pairs of virtues and vices. The vices are the major sickness-causing risk factors of our lives, whereas the virtues lead us back to health and wholeness.

In her fourth period, Hildegard undertook four extended mission trips up and down the Rhine and along the Main and Mosel Rivers. One can imagine the strain of these preaching tours on a woman over seventy years old. Her journeys often meant going by boat, on horseback, and on foot successively.

During this time (1163-1173), she wrote her last theological book *Liber Divinorum Operum*. In this *Book of Divine Works*, Hildegard describes humanity in the center of the cosmic circle as God's most complete creation. God forms humanity in the mother's womb; the workshop of God begins with conception. There is an exact description of the biochemical processes of the human body, which serves as an analogy to that which happens in the soul.

In her fifth period, shortly before her death, Hildegard dictated her autobiography to two monks. Unfortunately, the only personal work Hildegard wrote—as opposed to all her visionary works—exists today only as a fragment. When Hildegard died on the seventeenth of September, 1179, at the age of 81, a bright light glowed in heaven like a cross, a sign that she was able to see the living light. She, who once wrote the wonderful phrase, the "creation looks upon its creator like the beloved upon her lover," was now allowed to return home to the source of light.

With Hildegard's death, everything came to an end: her theology, prophecy, and medicine had no impact on the following generation whatsoever. Her medicinal book was not even included in *Corpus Hildegardicum* (1180-1190, Rupertsberg).

Hildegard never practiced medicine! As she testified herself: "I have never dedicated myself to the human studies of the learned." This is clearly evident from the total silence in all sources about any such practice. If she ever conducted studies or research, then at least some mention of such activity should be found, and yet none ever has. Her medicine would not be properly acknowledged for 800 years.

Why was it not until our century that Hildegard's medicine was discovered? We see that we are reaching a stage in medicine where our miraculous wonder drugs, like antibiotics and cortisone, are no longer effective against such disorders as allergies, multiple sclerosis, and AIDS. Out of God's wisdom, Hildegard medicine has perhaps been reserved for the helplessness of our times. It is so modern that only now, with our scientific knowledge of medicine, can we begin to appreciate Hildegard's remarkable understanding of the basic causes of health and sickness.

As proof and example of its absolutely modern scientific nature, let me mention two points. First, cancer is described so exactly in its origin and its manifestations that it has been a pleasure to see how the results of our modern cancer research have verified step by step what Hildegard describes. It is amazing to discover how Hildegard explains the precancerous state developing years before cancer is actually diagnosed. During this neglected period of precancer, Hildegard patients are treated preventatively, receiving an elixir to build up body resistance so that cancer is less likely to develop.

Second, Hildegard explains that detoxification is necessary in order to be healed. What is toxification of the body? He who thinks that nature gave men only remedies, and no poisons, is greatly in error! Strawberries, pork, and coffee, for example, are nutritional poisons. Environment, in the form of air pollution, food additives, or loud disco sound, can also be harmful. And finally, mental poisons like stress, distress, and anger change bile fluids, and thereby the chemistry of the blood.

Hildegard presents nearly 2000 remedies and health suggestions. There is a clearness in her presentation and a reason behind their use. Even today, no one is able to explain a single illness in the way Hildegard does. The most beautiful proof of all: her medicine works, it *does* heal!

In her last book on theology, Hildegard discloses the author of her book of medicine:

Everywhere in creation [trees, plants, animals, and precious stones] there are mysterious healing forces, which no person can know unless they have been revealed by God. (LDO I, 6, PL 893 C)

Hildegard calls the healing force itself *viriditas*. *Viriditas* literally mans greenness, growing energy, the principle of life and sexuality. Life from God transmitted into plants, animals, and precious stones is *viriditas*.

Hildegard medicine can be easily included in the large group of natural medicinal procedures which physicians can practice today. The difference between natural and modern medicine is that modern medicine is almost exclusively experimental medicine, whereas natural medicine leaves nature as it is. The rose is a rose; the apple tree has something unique about it; an orange is more than vitamin C.

Many people today feel this and are turning to natural healing methods. It will take a long time until we finally realize that nature has already made all the experiments. So we, too, can manage without experiments, which is not to say without experience. Having learned from experience, one returns to nature.

A new age is already beginning, and the shock that we are going through creates labor pains. Hopefully, a natural medicine may one day take its natural place. Hildegard's medicine stands or falls on its divine origin. In the light of historical research, we can say that any attempt to see her as a physician, or as a researcher in natural science, must fail miserably. The father of physicians, Hippocrates, once traced his profession back to divine ancestors. That was the world of the Greeks. To see Hildegard's medicine as coming from God, in the sense of a divine inspiration, is essentially the same thing.

What is new and basic in Hildegard's medicine? Hildegard's approach is comparable to the conviction of Paracelsus that all sickness must be curable, when he said that: "God does not allow a sickness to be unless there is also a remedy for it." We must only look. According to Hildegard, not cancer, but migraine and asthma are the most incurable illnesses. And cure here means a complete removal of the very roots, and not just the suppression of some symptoms.

I do not promise you immortality through Hildegard's natural treatment, but fullness of life, so that when you are "old and

144

filled with life" you can then take that great step into the everlasting state in full freedom and beauty. That, of course, requires a certain renunciation, e.g. of toxicating and addicting drugs, including tobacco and spirits (not wine, however)—and also coffee as your daily poison. Also you must have the courage to enter the proper relationship of doctor and patient, in that you gradually learn to be your own physician.

It is most important to take the responsibility for your own health. Enjoy a natural life and make proper use of your five senses. Take joy in walking, mountain-climbing, swimming, rowing, sailing, riding, fishing, taking care of animals, gardening, music and painting, etc. Believe in God, the essence of all good, creator and lord of the natural order of things.

Appendix A
REFERENCES

AP: *Aphorisms*

CC: *Causae et Curae* (part II of *Liber Compositae Medicinae,* or Book of Healing Methods)

LDO: *Liber Divinorum Operum* (Book of Divine Works)

LVM: *Liber Vitae Meritorum* (Book of Life's Merits)

PL: *Physica* (*Liber Simplicis Medicinae,* or Book of Composed Medicine)

SC: *Scivias* (Know the Ways, or Book of Faith)

Appendix B

CONVERSION TABLE

U.S./Metric Fluid Volume

1 teaspoon (tsp.) = ⅓ tablespoon = ⅙ fluid ounce = 5 milliliters = .005 liters

1 tablespoon (Tbsp.) = 3 teaspoons = ½ fluid ounce = ¹⁄₁₆ cup = 15 milliliters = .015 liters

1 fluid ounce (oz.) = 6 teaspoons = 2 tablespoons = ⅛ cup = ¹⁄₃₂ fluid quart = 29.56 milliliters = .030 liter

1 cup (c.) = 16 tablespoons = 8 fluid ounces = 236 milliliters = .236 liter

1 fluid quart (qt.) = 64 tablespoons = 32 fluid ounces = 4 cups = 946 milliliters = .946 liter

1 milliliter (ml.) = .203 or ⅕ teaspoon = .068 tablespoon = .034 fluid ounce = .004 cup = .001 liter

1 liter (l.) = 203.04 teaspoons = 67.68 tablespoons = 33.814 fluid ounces = 4.227 cups = 1.057 fluid quarts = 1000 milliliters

U.S./Metric Mass (Weight)

1 ounce (oz.) = 28.375 grams

1 gram (gm.) = .035 ounce

NOTE: European standards of measurement may differ slightly from those in the United States.

Appendix C
FURTHER INFORMATION ON HILDEGARD & HER PRODUCTS

Note that many of the Hildegard herbs and products are only recently becoming available in the United States. As more and more people become interested in her work, these products will become more readily available.

For further information about studies being done on Hildegard's work, contact:

The International Society of Hildegard von Bingen Studies
c/o Bruce W. Hozeski
Department of English
Ball State University
Muncie, IN 47306

ENGLISH / LATIN
BOTANICAL TABLE

agrimonia	*Agrimonia spp.*
aloe	*Aloe vera*
arum	*Arum maculatum*
basil	*Ocimum basilicum*
bay leaves (laurel)	*Laurus nobilis*
bedstraw	*Galium aparine*
burdock	*Arctium lappa*
camomile	*Anthemis nobilis*
caraway	*Carum carvi*
celery seed	*Apium graveolens*
chervil	*Anthriscus cerefolium*
cinnamon	*Cinnamomum zeylanicum*
clary sage	*Salvia sclarea*
cloves	*Caryophyllus aromaticus* or *Syzygium aromaticum*
columbine	*Aquilegia vulgaris*
cubeb cherries	*Piper cubeba*
cumin	*Cuminum cyninum*
cumin pimpernel	*Pimpinella saxifraga*
curled mint	*Mentha crispa*
dill	*Anethum graveolens*
duckweed	*Lemna minor*
English geranium	*Geranium anglicum*
euphorbia	*Euphorbia spp.*
fennel	*Foeniculum vulgare*
fenugreek	*Trigonella foenumgraecum*
field mint	*Mentha arvensis L*
field mustard	*Sinapis arvensis*
fleaseeds (psyllium)	*Plantago ovata*
galangal (catarrh root)	*Alpinia galanga* or *Alpinia officinalis*
ginger	*Zingiber officinale*
hart's tongue fern	*Scolopendrium vulgare*
herb robert	*Geranium robertianum*
horehound	*Marrubium vulgare*

149

horseradish	*Armoracia lapathifolia*
hyssop	*Hyssopus officinalis*
lavender	*Lavendula officinalis*
licorice	*Glycyrrhiza glabra*
linseed	*Linum usitatissimum*
long pepper	*Piper longum*
lovage	*Levisticum officinale*
lungwort	*Pulmonaria officinalis*
masterwort	*Imperatoria ostruthium*
mother of thyme	*Thymus serpyllum*
mugwort	*Artemisia vulgaris*
mullein	*Verbascum thapsus*
myrrh	*Commiphora myrrha*
nutmeg	*Myristica fragrans*
parsley	*Petroselinum sativum*
pellitory	*Anacyclus pyrethrum*
plantain	*Plantago spp.*
primrose	*Primula officinalis*
psyllium	*Plantago ovata*
quendal	*Herba serpylli*
quince	*Cydonia oblonga*
ribgrass (plantain)	(see plantain)
rose hip	*Rosa spp.*
rosemary	*Rosmarinus officinalis*
rue	*Ruta graveolens*
sage	*Salvia officinalis*
savory	*Satureja hortensis*
saxifrage	*Saxifraga spp.*
stinging nettles	*Urtica dioica*
tormentil	*Potentilla tormentilla*
valerian	*Valeriana officinalis*
vervain	*Verbena officinalis*
violet	*Viola spp.*
watercress	*Nasturtium officinale*
water mint	*Mentha aquatica*
wood betony leaves	*Stachys officinalis*
yarrow	*Achillea millefolium*
yellow gentian	*Gentiana lutea*
yew tree	*Taxus baccata*

NOTE: *spp. means "species"*

HILDEGARD LANGUAGE

DISCRETIO—The virtue of discretion. One of the personified virtues listed by Hildegard in *Liber Vitae Meritorum*.

DIVERSIS HUMORES—Noxious fluids.

GLAUBER'S SALT—Sodium sulphate, a bitter salt.

INFIRMI HUMORES—Infirm humor, or disease-related infectious juices.

JOCULATRIX—A craving for entertainment, one of the vices listed by Hildegard.

MALI HUMORES—Malicious humor, or bad juices.

MELANCHE—Black bile. See pages 36 and 77 for descriptions of its effects.

NOXI HUMORES—Noxious humor, or harmful juices.

SPELT—A grain, *Triticum spelta*, which has been cultivated and used as a source of food in Europe for over 6000 years. It is robust, allowing it to survive under extreme weather conditions, grow on the poorest soil, and live at altitudes which other wheat cannot tolerate. Spelt's edible kernal is surrounded by a tough, outer husk, which protects it from airborne pollutants, poisons, and radioactive fallout. As it has never been hybridized, spelt maintains an incredible degree of natural resistance, and requires no fertilizers, herbicides, or fungicides for cultivation. These characteristics, plus its superior nutritional properties, are the reasons for spelt's high recommendation by Hildegard.

VIRIDITAS—A Hildegard term, literally translated as "greening power," which forms a cornerstone for Hildegard's philosophy. She used it to refer to the life-force inherent in all of creation, the spirit by which all things grow, become fruitful, and celebrate the rich source of their life's power.

Appendix F

A NOTE
ON WHALE MEAT

During Hildegard's time (the twelfth century), whales were not considered to be the endangered species which they are today. Hildegard mentioned the use of whale meat in several of her dietary recommendations, which the editors felt ethically best to delete from the body of the book. For the sake of historical clarity, however, these deleted references are listed below:

Page 39. Whale was included in the list of seafoods to increase the intake of polyunsaturated fats.

Page 39. Whale was listed along with salmon as having the ability to lower cholesterol levels and prevent heart attacks.

Page 60. Under recommended meats, whale was mentioned as being "especially good for rheumatoid arthritis and gout."

INDEX OF
PLANTS & HERBS

nutmeg, 62, 84, 106
oats, 59, 111
onions, 60
oregano, 62
parsley, 35, 62, 111
peaches, 11, 64, 101
pears, 64
pellitory, 36, 37, 46, 62, 81, 136
pimpernel, 62
plantain, 31
plums, 64, 101
primrose, 82
psyllium, 49
pumpkin, 60
quendal, 136
quince, 60, 106
raspberries, 60
red beets, 60
ribgrass—see plantain
rose hip, 63
rosemary, 62

rue, 62, 106, 111, 123
rye, 59
sage, 20, 62, 123
savory, 62
saxifrage, 106
sinapis arvensis, 123
spelt, 44 ff., 58 ff., 136
stinging nettles, 40, 62
strawberries, 11, 64, 101 145
tormentil, 123
valerian root, 91
vervain, 16, 28
violet, 27, 129
watercress, 45, 60, 62
water mint, 62
wheat, 59, 112
white pepper, 36, 50, 53, 123
wood betony leaves, 89
yarrow, 126-127
yellow gentian, 38
yew-tree, 22
zittwer, 134

INDEX OF
SYMPTOMS & ILLNESSES

INDEX OF REMEDIES

ABOUT THE AUTHORS

Gottfried Hertzka, M.D. was born on October 12, 1913 in Bad Gastein, Austria. He grew up in Salzburg and graduated from the University of Vienna medical school. After the war he devoted his time to research and development of Hildegard's medicine, and later opened the Hildegard Practice in Konstanz. Encouraged by the results, he published several books on Hildegard's medicine and healing methods, including *So heilt Gott, Das Wunder der Hildegard-Medizin,* and *Die kleine Hildegard-Apotheke.* Dr. Hertzka is president of the German Hildegard society, *Forderkreis Hildegard von Bingen Sitz Konstanz am Bodensee.*

Wighard Strehlow, Ph.D. was born in Stettin on the Baltic Sea, grew up in East Germany, and graduated with a degree in natural science from Technical University in West Berlin. He continued his studies as a post-doctoral fellow at Yale University, and spent thirteen years in the German pharmaceutical industry. His initial research was on the synthesis and development of psychopharmaceuticals, antibiotics, and other drugs. He continued with clinical research, and finished his industrial career in acquisitions and licensing for natural healing products. In Konstanz, Dr. Strehlow met Dr. Hertzka and returned to his initial interest in natural science and holistic medicine. Since 1984 he has succeeded Dr. Hertzka at the Hildegard Practice in Konstanz. He is an active member of the Cooperation of Phytopharmaca, which registers Hildegard's medicinal plants for the German food and drug administration. He is married to Karin Anderson, who translated this book from German into English. They have two daughters and two sons.

BOOKS OF RELATED INTEREST
BY BEAR & COMPANY

ACCEPTING YOUR POWER TO HEAL
The Personal Practice of Therapeutic Touch
by Dolores Krieger, Ph.D., R.N.

BREATHING
Expanding Your Power & Energy
by Michael Sky

HILDEGARD OF BINGEN'S BOOK OF DIVINE WORKS
With Letters and Songs
edited by Matthew Fox

ILLUMINATIONS OF HILDEGARD OF BINGEN
text by Hildegard of Bingen
commentary by Matthew Fox

MEDITATIONS WITH HILDEGARD OF BINGEN
translated and adapted by Gabriele Uhlein

LIGHT: MEDICINE OF THE FUTURE
How We Can Use It to Heal Ourselves NOW
by Jacob Liberman, O.D., Ph.D.

VIBRATIONAL MEDICINE
New Choices for Healing Ourselves
by Richard Gerber, M.D.

Contact your local bookseller or write:
BEAR & COMPANY
P.O. Box 2860
Santa Fe, NM 87504